MW01533279

Love The Man
You Married

Angie Lewis

Heaven Ministries Press
South Carolina

Love The Man You Married

©2006 by Angie Lewis

First Printing

ISBN 1411677501
PRINTED BY Lulu Press
PUBLISHED BY
HEAVEN MINISTRIES
www.heavenministries.com

CONTENTS

Love The Man You Married

Love The Man You Married

How To Be Happy In Your Marriage
Introduction
1

A healthy marriage relies on the foundations of truth, honesty, honor, respect, and, above all, commitment. Couples don't have a problem staying married, that's the easy part! The difficult element of marriage is actually being happy and satisfied? Wouldn't you say? By honestly answering three questions, you will find out how to be happy in your marriage.

   1.) What is the purpose for your marriage?
   2.) What do you believe is truth for your marriage?
   3.) What do you believe in, and what do you believe for your marriage?

The conflict in many marriages of today is couples aren't making marriage a priority in their life; therefore, they have no real purpose to accomplish for the marriage. The solution is simple. Start making marriage more important in your belief system by doing those things for it that will help it to grow outward and flourish with abundance.

The obstacle facing couples here is the lack of the spiritual Christ surrounding the marriage. Couples tend to believe like the majority of society on what the virtues of marriage should be. Instead of basing the marriage upon a commitment of death do us part, they base it upon the lackadaisical attitude of "well if it turns out that I'm not happy in my marriage, I can always get a divorce."

But this kind of worldly thinking should not infuse our thoughts or we will always look for ways out of the relationship. The truth is, God was the great designer for marriage and couples should start basing that design into their own marriage.

The root of what we believe, our values and mores will ultimately steer us into the direction of our thoughts. For an example, if we believe it is ok to have sex outside of the marriage bed, then we will do those things that would ultimately steer us in that direction, and we'll, sooner or later, commit adultery. If we adhere to the worldly view of what "they" think is best for marriage, we'll end up following the wrong leader and make the wrong choices. Those choices steer us closer to divorce every single day. The wisdom we want for a healthy and productive marriage comes from God, not from what the world believes. God's wisdom for marriage is the indisputable truths we have been looking for. Now it is time to apply them into our own marriage. Why are they indisputable? Because we know that God's foundation already works for marriage, we know His truths are infallible and without a doubt the real deal.

Here is what one wife had to say. See if this hits home for any of you as well.

My husband and I are separated--not by my choice. I read your article called "Indisputable Truths for Marriage" and it is WONDERFUL! I even sent a copy to my husband and our pastor. I want my husband to see that divorce is not a right thing to do--and that just because things are hard doesn't mean that you just give up and throw the marriage away! We need to think about the legacy we

10

are starting for our children! I just can't say enough how your words affected my outlook today!!

Fortunately for her this wife found out that she doesn't want to end up like many couples of today; either divorced, separated or dreadfully unhappy in her marriage relationship with her husband. She has learned that true wisdom comes from God, and that is the direction she intends on steering her own marriage. The man who is looking to divorce this principled woman obviously doesn't know what he is missing out on because he will be losing an upright godly woman who has made her marriage a priority. Too bad he doesn't see it the same way.

Many of us choose marriage because we don't want to be alone in life. We want a lasting friendship/relationship with another to walk life's journey with. So what does that mean? It means husband and wife shouldn't go wondering off on separate roads, but stay together on the same roads learning and growing together. Marriage isn't always going to be beautiful roses, great sex, and nightly backrubs though. It takes a bit of spiritual effort to walk on the roads that lead to a happy marriage. It's knowing what you want and then doing it. It's knowing who you are and then being that person. Be real to your purpose in life. Don't try and be something that you're not. Marriage cannot take the adverse affects of a wishy-washy belief system. Marriage thrives on stability. If husband and wife are walking on separate roads the marriage is going to have problems, plain and simple. Are you in the boat with your husband or are you in your own boat?

Many times walking on the same roads requires that we compromise with each other; giving up something YOU enjoy for the sake of YOUR husband. This is how you bring happiness and contentment into the marriage. So what is the purpose for your marriage? Only you can answer that but if it involves God in the picture then you will eventually come to find that purpose. God wants you to find your purpose. If you're not with your husband now, get back in the boat with him and seek your purpose for your marriage together. Give your marriage the importance it deserves!

I do know that choosing happiness and satisfaction is important in most people's lives, is it not? It is something we all want. Who doesn't want to be happy? How will you attain this happiness? What will you do to bring happiness into your marriage for your self and husband? It takes a little bit of effort. In all reality, sometimes it takes a whole lot of effort. But that is why you got married, right? Didn't you say that you would love your man through the good times and the bad? You knew it wasn't going to be a bed of roses all the time. Sometimes there's going to be some thorns. If we seek God's truth for marriage those thorns will turn into a bed of cotton, believe me.

You can't really expect your husband to make you happy twenty four-seven? Isn't this asking too much of him? If you require inner peace from another human being it isn't going to happen. So the answer to what your purpose is then is simple, really, you just need to turn the tables around. Your purpose for marriage is for YOU to bring the happiness, and satisfaction into play for both you and your husband to enjoy, instead of relying upon or expecting him to do it for both of you. Somebody's got to do it! Why not you? You'll do it when you decide your marriage is important to YOU.

So what does this mean? It means giving out a little bit more of your self than you already have, and doing it, even when you don't feel like it. That little bit more of something might be learning and studying the Bible more or it just might be staying home on girl's night out because your husband wants you to help him with some paperwork. Whatever the little bit more of oneself that you do give, just be happy that you are married to the man you are married to. Your attitude will change instantly just by changing your thought patterns.

So what if you do most of the giving, you shouldn't be keeping score or you will never be happy. Keeping score keeps us under the bondage of our negative feelings and we don't want that.

Love The Man You Married

Because you are married, you have a big job ahead of you, but it is an important task that should never be overlooked. It is such an important responsibility that not everyone can do it. In fact, most people choose to live under the control of their feelings and they remain unhappy and unsatisfied. That is why there is so much divorce circulating around in this country. Most people choose to look out into the culture of society for their marriage answers and look where that is getting them.

I think it would be fair to say that when you said your vows while looking into your husbands eyes, you intended on making him happy, didn't you? Remember this is part of the reason you married him, right, to bring happiness into the marriage for both of you? Nothing has changed from when you were first married up to now, so go after your purpose, and remember it is not to be taken lightly.

So what do you believe is truth for your marriage? The selfish way of believing is living in the "I want mode" of thinking. This selfish pattern girdles on what you believe. Culture of society plays itself out with this kind of thinking. People are like chameleons, individuality is lost, and becomes one in its beliefs. A corrupt culture is formed through spiritual bankruptcy. It flourishes on selfish thinking and rebelliousness to the truth.

The bottom line is this. You have choices for your marriage, choose wisely, grab onto who you are, and stay in the same boat with your husband while you *both* paddle towards the same purpose. Don't let the waves bring you down; you have Gods' indisputable truths for support.

You're not the only one who walks away from God and towards the world for support of their marriage. Fortunately, some of you have woken from your slumber and have found your self. One of my newsletter readers finally got it all figured out and then emailed me to tell me the great revelation. And I'm glad she did.

I just wanted to let you know that I'm amazed by the fact that I have seen 2 different counselors over the past few years and one immediately wanted to put me on anti-depressant medication (which I opted not to do) and the other was steering me down the "do whatever it takes...everyone will survive with or without one another" path. And the advice you have given me over just the past month is what is hitting home and making sense! I even spent 4 days (24 hrs total) attending a long weekend seminar about "waking up and finding yourself" and that didn't even work. I've read 3 of your newsletter articles found in the Heaven Ministries website and can relate to and understand what you are trying to teach people. The hard part is putting it all into real life play! Just another little thanks to YOU! Again, I'll keep in touch as progress is made and, or if I'm stuck and can't move.

It's True. At some point in time, we will get stuck and feel we cannot get out of the rut we're in and this is the perfect time to come out from the negative feelings we're so used to wallowing in and look into God's indisputable truths.

Sometimes in marriage we women might only care about our own happiness and leave our husband to take care for himself. It's normal; I used to do it all the time with my own husband. But this is selfish, and it is this kind of thinking that believes that spending a bunch of money and getting more stuff will bring us the happiness that is missing from marriage. After all, our husband's aren't doing anything to make us happy so maybe a long drawn out shopping spree we'll make us happy.

This is how we ladies think sometimes. Believe me I have done my share of shopping, only to feel guilty about it later. What does all the stuff we buy do for our marriage? Absolutely nothing!

The power of happiness and satisfaction lies within what we can do for our self, that's all! "Things" don't make us happy and neither do riches. Happiness is within the person we are and it's up to us to bring forth that happiness in any way in which we can. Go for it!

Love The Man You Married

"Keep your lives free from the love of money and be content with what you have, because God has said, "Never will I leave you; never will I forsake you" Hebrews 13:5

If you are feeling dissatisfied or discontented in your marriage it is because there is something drastically missing in your life; you're just not sure what that missing piece is. Many women believe the discontent of their marriage to mean, they are no longer in love with their husband, and so their *thinking* makes them stop loving their husbands the way they are supposed to love them. But what's really missing are beliefs built upon the foundations of godly wisdom, love and truth. It is not that you have stopped loving your husband; it is that you have literally stopped loving your husband! Your beliefs have created a way of life that feeds off self to survive. But, believe me, you cannot love or give of your self properly if you are living off of self-based love.

The greatest goal and purpose you can attain for your marriage should to be more loving! To be more giving! To love not on demand or with strings attached, but to just love. We accomplish this goal by handing over the selfish person we are now to God and letting Him take over for us in the selfish department. Once this is done, we can learn to love others with freedom by giving of ourselves with no strings or demands attached. ♥

Love The Man You Married

2

"Love is patient, love is kind. It does not envy, it does not boast, it is not proud. It is not rude, it is not self-seeking, it is not easily angered, it keeps no records of wrongs. Love does not delight in evil but rejoices with truth. It always protects, always trusts, always hopes, always preserves."
1 Corinthians 13:4-7

I believe the word "love" is thrown around just a bit too nonchalantly. Don't you think? People say they love but do nothing to SHOW that love. Love needs action to complete its purpose. So when I say "love who you married" that means to provide of your self in the marriage. That *is* what love is all about.

Let's take a look at 6 biblically based principles that make up several areas of loving.

16

Love The Man You Married

1. Love Is Patient!

Are you patient with your husband? Patience is a virtue. It is a wonderful character trait to have and practice patience. Are you utilizing all of the potential that God has given you? Are you patient, or are you easily irritated and annoyed? Do you really listen to what your husband has to say or do you not show interest and keep busy doing something else as he talks? Are you considerate and understanding of your husbands needs? Being patient with your man is one way you can furnish love to him.

2. Love Does Not Envy!

Are you jealous of the man you married? Do you ever envy or resent your husband? Resentment runs rampant in marriages today, and it is literally tearing couples apart! You don't want resentment to tear apart your marriage, do you? So often I hear couples tell me how resentful they are of their spouse for one reason or another, but mostly over petty little things that only need to be discussed! Instead what are they doing? Getting even! Have you talked to your husband today?

Here is what one husband said about his marriage with his wife of twenty years. When I received his email, I immediately emailed him back and told him about the people pleaser personality. I told him to start writing down the times his wife felt guilty for not being available to others, and to sit down with her right then and there and properly discuss the situation. I believe that his wife really needs to do more things for her self. She is so unhappy that she is having are hard time trying to please anyone else, mostly her poor husband! Here is what he had to say. See if you can glean anything useful out of it.

My wife and me have been married for 20 yrs. About 3 weeks ago she stopped showing me affection. I'm not talking about sex. I confronted her about it and she said everything is bothering her. Her dad has Lou

Gehrig's disease and her mother makes her feel guilty when we go away for a weekend. She also said she doesn't know if she has the right kind of love for me anymore. She also said she has been harboring pain for 20 years-- funny she didn't show it. She goes to church every Sunday, and I have been going back lately. I have never cheated on her. I told her I would not cheat. Any ideas?

What do you think about this husband's situation? Can you just for a moment put your self in his shoes? This is what I try to do when I receive painful cries for help. It is so sad and I think that if I can try and put myself in the individual's situation I can see the picture more clearly. Do you think his wife is resentful of him/parents/marriage/life? I do. She has been harboring negative feelings towards her husband, and for a long time!

This is one of the main reasons for not showing affection to you husband. Are the feelings of resentment stopping you from feeling any loving affection for the man you married?

When I put my self in the other person's shoes, not only can I understand the picture more clearly but I can see myself in the picture as well. Not now, mind you, but several years ago, I too, was in the situation as his wife, and my poor husband was the one left out in the cold to deal with my often moody and negative emotional disposition.

As you can see, her thoughts are controlling her ability to love her husband properly. Unfortunately this woman doesn't know how to stop letting her negative emotions and thoughts control her marriage. Hopefully with the right self expression and biblical applications this man can help his wife to learn to start doing things for her self, stop people pleasing, and learn to love him again, properly.

3. Love Is Not Self-Seeking!!
This is a biggy in marriage! I talk quite a bit about selfishness in my book, *Journey on the Roads Less Traveled*, and also in many of my articles off my website. Why? I believe this to be a major issue with couples in marriages

today even though it doesn't always seem apparent. I do know from experience how a selfish spouse can tear the other down with them. I've been there and done that once upon a time in my own marriage. In the first years of my marriage I was so "into myself", and so out in left field for my marriage, that is, until I found the love of Jesus for my life. That's all it took for me. It took God to come first in my life.

We all have some selfish qualities that we shine intensely on occasion, but some of us are so selfish in marriage that we don't know how to give of our self at all!! Many issues cause selfish behavior, but mostly it is lack of the spiritual Christ intervening within our inner being. We're trying to lead our life under our own understanding instead of allowing the spirit within us to work out the daily issues that affect us.

What we allow into our mind is what we will output onto others; mainly to the person we married. This is why I stress so often in my newsletter and articles that for a healthy and sound marriage couples need to take care of them selves *first*, then and only then, can they help the marriage.

What are you allowing into your mind? Beliefs from the world often corrupt marriage and turn it into something ugly and immoral.

4. Love Is Not Easily Angered!

Do you get angry with your husband over nothing! Do you ever think that you might be behaving impatient and intolerable with your husband? What underlying problem might be charging your anger? If you are quick to anger, then it could be that something deeper is bothering you. Until you get to the root of your anger it will remain within your inner psyche ready to emotionally abuse whoever gets in the way. If you are abusing your husband with your angry feelings, leave the house if you have to. It is wrong to berate your husband with bad feelings of anger. In your anger you might say and do things that you normally wouldn't. Your angry words can bruise his ego, especially if this emotional abuse is continuous.

"My dear brothers, take note of this: Everyone should be quick to listen, slow to speak and slow to become angry, for man's anger does not bring about the righteous life that God desires." James 1:19-20

"A hot-tempered man stirs up dissension, but a patient man, calms a quarrel." Proverbs 15:18

5.   Love Does Not Delight In Evil but Rejoices In Truth! This has to be the champion of all the aspects of love because if we followed this one simple principle we would not need any other standards to tell us how to love, or what love is. This straightforward verse speaks for itself, but for some of you, maybe you are not sure what the truth is. The truth is what will set you free from all of the above unpleasant aspects of your character, such as anger, resentment, envy, jealousy and strife. After all, these are only feelings that you carry around inside your head. You can either make them your life or find a new way of life. If you want to be free of these feelings you need to find the truth, right? You need to *know* the truth, right?

Bottom line is the truth not only sets us free from negative feelings that might be controlling our life, but will also make us new people within that truth. Once we start applying the truth into our life is when we can easily stop carrying around any bitter feelings, and negative attitudes that we may have. Simply said, truth is God's words of wisdom; therefore, we will be walking in truth when we apply God's truth into our life.

The woman who has wisdom is loving towards her husband, is faithful, honest, trustworthy, committed, trusts in

Love The Man You Married

God, puts God first, turns away from evil, knows right from wrong, listens and learns, and applies wisdom into all areas of her life.

"Long life is in her right hand; in her left hand are riches and honor. Her ways are pleasant ways and all her paths are peace. She is a tree of life to those who embrace her; those who lay hold of her will be blessed." Proverbs 3:13-18

And that is the truth! Do you have the wisdom to love the man you married? ♥

Biblical Precepts For Your Marriage
3

S ometimes in marriage we just need to hear it again. We need to hear that marriage takes a few simple guidelines to help it along. With time we tend to forget that our marriage needs a bit of Tender Loving Care once in while. Because of this, I have made a list of a few areas I think all marriages could utilize to bring back that punch that is so vital in marriage. Husbands should read, study and utilize these aspects of marriage as well. Type them out and put them up on the refrigerator for daily discussion and application.

1) Communicate feelings effectively for spiritual growth. By expressing feelings appropriately we learn to be honest with who we are. Expressing ourselves properly is a growth process that takes time and the willingness to allow issues to come out in a good way rather than wallowing in resentment or exploding with anger.

2) Women who understand themselves and utilize their inner spirit have better marriages. This is so true! What can you do to better understand the wife you are and the person you are? Learn to listen and recognize the positive aspects of who you are, which is the spiritual side and apply those things into the marriage.

3) Wives who respect the role of their husbands and allow them to be captain of the ship find its sails steering into many blessings at the shore.

4) Husbands who respect the role of the wife as being the helpmate and co-worker within marriage find it flourishes with abundance and the marriage develops and is happy.

5) Wives who allow their husbands the freedom to be themselves find they are less stressful and more caring and giving. Even though husband and wife become one in body when they are married, couples still have their individual personality traits that make them who they are.

6.) Forgive by letting go of resentment. This is why we cannot forgive past issues; resentment and bitter hearts keep us from forgiving those we love the most. Believe me about resentment. It is a bad thing to carry around in your heart.

7) Couples who pray together stay together. Read, study, and apply the biblical foundations into your marriage.

8) Shift your man-made foundation into a spiritual supported one when dealing with marital issues. The world is not going to help your marriage. In fact it will break it in two very fast.

9) Learn to use your God given talents positively in marriage. Some of us have so much energy and we waste it on bickering and blaming instead of looking for ways to use that energy in the positive for our marriage.

10) Humble yourselves to each other. This means there is no need to get in the last word or to always be right. You don't have to be wrong either, but when you give in, you become right for doing what is right for the marriage. Giving in during arguments instead of wasting time fussing and fighting is the way to be meek and modest. Even if you are right, it certainly isn't worth the conflicts it brings into the marriage, right?

The power of a woman's words, by what she says and how she says it becomes a learned "way of behaving" and if those words are negative they will eventually break down the structural integrity of the relationship. Following a set of precepts will help us to remember that.

A great marriage involves team players working towards the good of the relationship. This is what "team work" is all about. We should help pull together the area in the relationship where our husband is less practiced then we are. This way the marriage is complimented by each other's ideas, goals and working environment. I realize that most of the time, we women are a bigger team players when it comes down to working together, but we're good at it, and so play well when we want to.

When we do little things for our husband, instead of complaining about it, it takes some of the stress off of him. We need to keep our husbands organized and focused ladies! We shouldn't fight with him, and try to take charge, or control him. We want the marriage to grow and flourish, and it will, if we put forth that extra effort to work together as a team even if that means we women end up doing more for the marriage. We certainly don't want to dominate our husbands, do we? No! We want the marriage to be one institution, not two institutions fighting over who is going to be in charge.

Love The Man You Married

Of course, we can always try and take the easy way out and continually harass and pick and peck at our husband as we try to take the splinter out of his eye. But it won't do a bit of good, until we take the log out of our own first.

It is by realizing our own actions and how WE can change, that we actually see clearly enough to react in beneficial ways toward our husband when marital issues do occur.

Love the man you married. ♥

Submit To The Man You Married

4

I sincerely believe myself to be a freer, happier and more content-filled woman than those who strive so hard to be something they really aren't. Face it, women weren't meant to control the world of men, just like men were not meant to wear a bra and pantyhose.

Don't get me wrong, there is nothing at all wrong with a successful career minded woman, but if it takes away from the obvious responsibilities that a woman was meant to partake in, then it is absolutely not acceptable.

The truth of the matter is these particular women only want to be validated for who they are. But who are they? I don't even think they know who they are! They must define them self through a means that makes them feel better about themselves. Their resentment towards men makes them feel better when they are behaving like men in high heels.

All of this unnecessary hoopla stems from the emotional imbalance of the spiritual self. Unfortunately, while these women strive to be the TOTAL woman, their particular issues and causes go against the desire of the Creator, and their spirit stays out of whack and out of tune with the normal responsibilities inherited within them from when they were created.

For some reason when they achieve the things that go against their very nature of womanhood is when they feel validated? In retrospect all of this originates from how they feel about themselves and as women. Ironically, these women validate each other through wrong thinking. They don't understand that their own negative feelings towards being a woman actually control the real woman they can become. They are wasting their potential as women, and because of that, loving, caring husbands, and children are suffering because of it!

The real issue here is when a woman tries to define her being (soul) through the act of abortion or the act of leadership and power, she is actually in rebellion to God when her spirit should be tending to the necessities of children, husband, and home life.

A woman doesn't have to be brow beaten, manhandled or treated like a mat because she submits to her husband!! This sort of thinking is way out in left field on what submission truly means!

I am an extremely independent woman and found your article on submission to be amazing. I was a teen bride and then remarried in my early 20's. That also failed. Now at 36, I am newly engaged and am in complete agreement with every word that was spoken in your article!

For years I attempted to be 'equal' to my mate. It is only recently that I fully understand the Divine meaning of Christ wanting to have my helpmate lead and for us to go forth together. I know the reason it took me so long was due to my upbringing,, the horrible childhood and a past that haunted me. I am very pleased to say the Lord brought my fiancée and I together. He is God fearing, he wants to please our Father and me, he will not 'abuse' the fact that I completely submit to him. I know I can, because I trust him with my life.

Wow! Now this woman calls herself extremely independent and said she *knows* she can completely submit to her husband because she trusts him. The missing link to submission is all about trust! The bottom line is, we trust our husbands because we trusted in God first.

In all reality, it is not in a woman's true nature to lord over men. I don't really think they want to be the leader in the home but for some reason, probably lack of communication, and the need to control every aspect of the home, it just ends up being that way. Couples aren't talking about their marital issues anymore instead they are separating and getting divorced!

But still, I don't understand why some of these women can't see where the milk comes from. Pardon the pun. Women are leaders in their own right! They are selected in doing what they do best, nurturing babies, bringing up loving and respectful children, being beautiful, inside and out, keeping him organized and focused, and supporting him. This is leading! Our man needs us, ladies. He needs us to be the woman in his life.

There is no family without the woman. The woman is the main linkage of the family. She is the connection that keeps it all together, and flowing smoothly, if she wants it to. She is the nurturer and lover. She is the one who brings peace and comfort into the home. It is not degrading to be a woman; it is degrading trying to be a man in high heels!

A married woman certainly can't do a very good job taking care of her husband if she is out trying to conquer the world of men. Right?

As we all know, the bible says the wife should submit to her husband's spiritual authority and the husband should love the wife? What does it mean?

The husband should love is wife so he can offer his spiritual authority properly. If a man doesn't love his wife properly, then he probably can't give acceptable spiritual counsel either, wouldn't you agree?

If a husband loves his wife, then he is going to make sure that nothing harms her. He will protect her as much as he possibly can. He might not want her to drive at night by herself in the car. He might not want her to wear a skimpy bikini to the beach when he is not with her. He might not want her to spend time with friends who really aren't friends, but are bad influences. He might not want her to work outside of the home, because he feels that it is his responsibility to take care of his family financially.

None of those things above are because a husband doesn't necessarily trust his wife but because he doesn't want his wife subjected to the consequences of those actions. In this society I sometimes wonder while I'm watching the nightly news on TV, what man in his right mind would allow his wife to go out alone at night, unless it is absolutely necessary. I mean, women are getting beaten, shot, raped, and murdered quite frequently in our local Wal-Mart store parking lots!

Do you think that submitting to your husband makes you inferior to him, and not in control of your womanhood? Well it is not true. When a woman allows her Christ-honoring husband to lead the household she is putting her faith in God, and respecting the role of her husband as well. This is real validation!

When a husband orders that his wife submit to him, then it's not true submission. Taking advantage of scripture and using it out of context as a mere tool for intimidating and hurting your wife is wrong and leads to resentment. There is no application in this instance.

But this is precisely why God says that a husband should love his wife like Christ does the church! A Christ-honoring man is a man who loves his wife, and he will not take advantage of his leadership role. Likewise, a Christ-honoring wife will not try to undermine her husband's leadership role. It's really that simple.

Husbands are to love their wives, and ladies we are to submit to that love! Come on ladies, giving in to the authority of your husband doesn't mean you have lost your rights as a woman or individuality. It doesn't mean that you are not independent minded enough to think on your own and have your own opinions either. What it means is you love and respect your husband for being a man! What is so wrong with that? Submission is being respectful. Just as the wife submits to her husband so should the husband to the Lord.

Let's look at it another way and pretend that this scripture was never written.

There is only one captain to every ship and with that ship there is only one first mate. The captain needs his first mate, she is the one who reads the navigational charts and brings out the sails and brings in the lines. She is there for him when storms come and waves are washing up onto the deck. She cooks for him to bring him energy during the storm because while she is sleeping, he is still steering the ship through the storm to safety.

The husband is the helmsman and the wife is the first mate. What a wonderful relationship. The first mate is supportive, caring, and helpful beyond belief. Without the first mate to lend a hand in times of need and decision-making, the ship would sink.

The first mate needs the captain for without a captain to steer the ship, there would be no destination-no purpose to why you were together in the first place.

If both the captain and the first mate try and take the helm and lead the ship to separate shores, the ship ends up adrift because both are steering in separate directions.

So ladies, when we rebel against our husband's divine authority, we are actually rebelling against the will of God.

The bottom line: Someone has to be the head of the family, and in nature, history and scripture that somebody has always been the male. God gives him this position not of demanding ruler-ship, but of responsibility and honor. So to the men who are reading this, love your wives with the WISDOM God gave you and she will submit out of her enduring love for you! ♥

How To Forgive an Adulterous Husband

5

Have you tried to forgive your husband of adultery only to have it all come back to haunt you later? This happens because we have not forgiven in its completeness. Anyone can say they have forgiven, but what is your heart telling you?

Do you think it is the end of your marriage because your husband had an affair? On the contrary it's time to nurture, cultivate, and cherish the marriage even more. It is time to start plucking out the mischievous weeds to make room for the tender new shoots.

The purpose for forgiving those who have hurt us is to clear out unwanted emotions, and free our minds from negative clutter. This needless stuff builds up if we don't do anything about it. First and foremost we need to be mentally and spiritually healthy so we can express feelings and needs appropriately to our husband. Then and only then can we actually forgive in completeness?

One of the most difficult aspects of forgiving is the ability to stop picturing the hurt in our mind. We may actually try and envision what it was like for our husband while he was engaged in the sexual act with another women. We want to know if he enjoyed it or not. We want to know why he did it. We may even believe there is something wrong with us sexually. All of these things enter our mind even after we have forgiven, and they can literally tear us apart.

My motto has always been that we absolutely need to take care of our self first before we can take care of another. If we are all messed up inside, full of bitterness and resentment towards our unfaithful husband, we certainly cannot forgive him properly. The same applies with love. Don't we need to love ourselves first before we can love another?

So this brings me to detachment. We become healthy in mind by detaching with love. What's that? As Jesus would say, "Turn the other cheek." We need to let it go! Letting emotional qualms trouble us will not help the forgiveness process. When we let the anger and bitterness go from within our inner being, we can start applying constructive ways to build back up our wounded marriage.

Detaching only means we are not going to allow the weakness of our husband to control our mental and spiritual well-being. If we are still angry and bitter over their unfaithfulness, we invariably make their sin a part of who we are by obsessing over it every chance we get. Detaching gives us the freedom to forgive!

If we refuse to forgive our husband we are missing out on the wonderful opportunity to experience the joys in forgiving and sharing that happiness with the man we married. The marriage will miss out on the growth process that takes place within its framework, and our own spiritual outlook on life. Marriage can remain stunted by not forgiving or we can finally begin to grow out from the selfish person we have been by forgiving our husbands of their sin against the marriage, and doing it with completeness of our heart.

No doubt, it is difficult to forgive when we think of our

husbands in bed with someone else. But that's just it; we are flabbergasted that he would err against the marriage in such a way. We feel duped, unloved, and deceived! We want restitution at all costs! For some of us that means divorce. This initial feeling, of course, is completely understandable. We have been hurt deeply by the unfaithfulness of our husband and justify our own bad behavior by literally making ourselves the victim of our husband's weakness. But who really is the victim here? At some point and time we absolutely need to forgive or else we persecute ourselves with our own hurt emotions.

In reality, we make our self the victim of our husband's sin by obsessing over it and not forgiving. We do that to our self. No one does that for us. Divorce over unfaithfulness is totally unnecessary. Couples can work through this infidelity issue properly and grow from it to boot.

Do you think your husband had an affair to do wrong purposely against the marriage or you? I don't believe this to be true. Most of the time when a husband is unfaithful it has nothing to do with the wife, even though they like to finger point and blame. The reasons behind unfaithfulness stem from the need for constant self-gratification, low self esteem, and lack of spiritual wisdom and knowledge. Having a not so good marriage does not give anyone the right to commit the act of adultery. God has given us other useful tools that we can bring into the marriage when the issues of adultery come into play. Divorce is unnecessary.

Here's how it usually works. First the idea to be unfaithful is imagined in the mind. Secondly it is mediated on with vivid scenes and great clarity. Thirdly, the act of adultery somehow becomes justified because of wrong thinking taking over because of cultural influences. Finally the act of adultery is actually carried out in the physical sense. Sometimes the guilty party feels remorse about defiling the marriage bed, and won't do it again. No one finds out, case closed.

But sometimes-promiscuous acts continue, and that is because the unfaithful husband has not humbled him self to

God for the guidance he so very much needs to help him to turn away from tempting and enticing situations. Unfaithfulness in marriage is only a symptom of a greater problem. But so often when marriages break apart couples blame infidelity as the culprit, but it is not the real problem.

The real issue is most likely boredom, lack of respect and commitment for one another. But those are the main features God had designed especially for marriage! And since the culture of society has made it justifiable to sleep around from bed to bed, house to house, couples have decided to make themselves a part of that promiscuous world instead of God's world. So in essence the real problem stems from lack of spiritual wisdom guiding couples in their faithless marriage!

Unfortunately, so many marriages of today deal with the issue of adultery. Culturally speaking, isn't it a thing of normalcy for a spouse to be unfaithful in their marriage? No one gives a darn! But this kind of thinking is destroying lives. It is not normal to have sexual relations outside of marriage! It is very wrong and goes against all that God has created and planned for marriage! Adultery breaks the bonds of trust and respect for the person we married, and carries with it a heavy sword of sinful rebellion against what God has created.

You see, if we have not yet acknowledged the realm of God's world and are lacking in the knowledge of God's goodness, we, through our own understanding, allow our wayward thinking patterns to take charge. But what do we know? We know our negative feelings! That's what we know.

Our feelings tell us to be bitter because our husband had sex with someone else. So what do we do? We become bitter! Our feelings tell us to stay resentful, and so we resent him! Our feelings tell us the grass is greener over there on the other side of the fence. So we go to the other side. How can we forgive properly when our negative feelings our controlling us! These unhealthy emotions make our attitude, and ultimately tell us how to view the world around us and how to live in the world.

A healthy spiritually minded woman allows her self to be

directed by God's insight where it looks beyond selfishness and into the loving person she was meant to be. We absolutely need to have the knowledge and wisdom of God within the framework of who we are, so we can understand how to respect and love our husband properly. Love the man you married? Get off the sand and build your house on the rock.

In Matthew it tells us, "Therefore everyone who hears these words of mine and puts them into practice is like a wise man who built his house on a rock. The rain came down, the streams rose and the winds blew and beat against that house; yet it did not fall, because it had its foundation on the rock. But everyone who hears these words of mine and does not put them into practice is like a foolish man who built his house on sand. The rain came down, the streams rose, and the winds blew and beat against the house, and it fell with a great crash." Matthew 7:24-27

One repentant man wrote in to me addressing a certain article I wrote on the topic of forgiving a spouse of adultery. Here is what he had to say about how he felt after committing the act of adultery. His wife would not forgive him and she was literally tormenting him with all her unforgiveness and rotten emotions.

Your article on forgiveness was very comforting. After cheating on my wife, I felt so helpless and worthless. I would do anything to go back and change what happened and there's nothing I can do. My wife will not forgive me, and she torments me continuously about my mistake, it wears at my innermost being. The sorrow and grief and shame are unbearable. I could not think of a better gift and proof of true love and character than forgiving someone that has hurt you, especially someone who has hurt you deeply. I hope to experience this gift one day and be able to have a full heart once again.

Bottom line: The ability to forgive does not stand with us alone. We just do not have the complete understanding to actually forgive without ever bringing up the offense again to our husband, and even to our self! What happens is we only forgive superficially, which keeps us feeling the burden of the hurt. But we don't want this because here is what happens. If we only forgive superficially the offense will continually evade our heart and mind like the poor woman above, and consequently bitter feelings will take over and control what we do and how we behave.

Do you want to lash out in anger at your husband? Then forgive superficially. Do you want to say hateful and mean things to the man you married? Then forgive superficially. Do you want to respect and trust your husband again? Then forgive completely.

Here is how we forgive. First, understand this: The Holy Spirit is our greatest blessing and gift from God that we, as His children receive when we share ourselves with Him. When we give up the selfish ego to God, He will in return gives us the gift of how to love properly, how to hope, how to have faith with conviction, and how to forgive completely. When we act on His instructions we are allowing the power of the Holy Spirit to take over in our marriage and life and we are submitting to His will for us.

God is in control. Remember, we do not have the ability under our own understanding to forgive properly, to love completely, or to understand and utilize the blessed gifts of the Holy Spirit. We know that all these awesome gifts come from God. But that is all we know. Not until we put all of this into practice will it actually be real to us. We will not understand what it is that God wants for us, until we submit our sinful and selfish lives to Him. We want it all. But to have it, we must experience God's forgiveness for us first. ❤

I Can't Forgive My
Cheating Husband!
6

I am tormenting my husband everyday because he had an affair. I wish that I could stop abusing him, but I can't, it hurts so badly sometimes. I know it is wrong of me to treat him with so much cruelty, but I just can't help it. I keep picturing him in bed with that woman! What can I do?

Why do you think this woman is not forgiving her husband? She thinks she is benefiting from using her negative feelings against her husband. She is allowing the hurt she feels to control her thoughts about her husband to such a degree that she is using this power over her husband to make her self feel better, and the funny things is, it works! It is so true. She might feel better for about five minutes until her unforgiving heart needs fed again. She will envision her husband in bed with another woman and then abuse her husband with it every chance she gets. This is how she deals with the pain.

Those of us who have dealt with the issue of adultery can relate to this woman's wounded heart but what about her husband? What happens to him? What is he supposed to do for the pain he is feeling?

Not everyone can forgive properly but without true forgiveness, the marriage will be threatened by lack of trust, which only a spiritual perceptiveness can repair. With that said, this woman can either continue wallowing in her pain or come out from her selfish feelings she is now living in and decide to forgive her husband.

So lets look at this issue a bit closer. The wife is hurting, "big time" over her husband's stupid and sinful mistake but he is remorseful and asking for forgiveness. Therefore, this woman needs to stop living inside of her feelings, and come out of her selfishness and start taking care of her marriage before there is no marriage left to take care of! Wouldn't you agree? I know, I sound pretty strong with some of these people, but someone has to tell them. Bing! Reality! Come down out of that fluffy cloud you're on. Marriage counselors aren't saying anything because they don't want to rock the boat, or else couples will go to a different marriage counselor.

The day after I wrote this article I had a lady email me about how much this particular article helped her to see how selfish she was being in her own marriage. So you see how a little nudge from a supportive stranger helps? Here is what she said.

I just finished reading your article and I thank you for it. My husband cheated on me several times then came and confessed to me. He cried his heart out to me because he felt so bad. He has apologized almost everyday since I put him out in October of 2004. I was so hurt myself, that until I read your article today I never thought about the pain he must be feeling. Our 6th anniversary is this month. He has been asking me to come home for over 11 months now. I now know what I will give him for our anniversary, thanks to you. I am going to give him a new start on our marriage, back where he belongs. Here at home with me, his wife. Thank you for showing me how selfish I was.

I am so thrilled to know that some of these women are finally coming around and not allowing their marriage to be destroyed completely over the act of adultery.

What can a wife do to help her to forgive her husband of adultery? She needs to realize that it doesn't CHANGE anything by NOT forgiving. The time and energy wasted on an unforgiving heart is utterly useless. She cannot turn back the clocks here and pretend it didn't happen. She needs to let the pain finally go by forgiving.

Granted, you can never forget the past, but that doesn't mean you cannot learn to forgive completely either, which is essentially not abusing your husband with it every darn chance you get. It is quite normal for a wife to be angry, bitter, and resentful towards her husband after he had an affair, and it's perfectly okay for her to get those feelings out of her system. Even if that means to scream, shout, and name call. All of these feelings and actions are all very normal—for a time. And only for a time!

Eventually, after the initial shock is over, ask God to help relieve the pain from within you and learn to stop the verbal abuse. No marriage can last for very long when one spouse is abusing another mentally and emotionally.

In marriages that aren't so great to begin with, adultery is used as a weapon to manipulate and control the adulterer with. It is a strong weapon, wielded at the most opportune times to feel better about self, to get what you want, to seem like the good guy, and sometimes to destroy the marriage through divorce. But none of this is necessary. I know this because I have been there and done that. I have been on both sides of this issue. Both sides are filled with heartache and despair but it can be rectified through the proper foundations.

We are all human beings and make mistakes but God knows in our heart that if we are remorseful of our mistakes, He will give us a chance to ask for His forgiveness. Of course we need time to reflect, and to lament, and to even dwell on the hurt we are feeling but we cannot go on living on that foundation or the marriage will definitely fall.

We have to be willing to make amends and to forgive our husband with the same forgiveness that God has forgiven us with?

Jesus says we are to forgive the adulterer *if* they have stopped in their weakness and have repented. We have all sinned. Is this woman better than her husband because she wasn't the one caught in the act of adultery? I don't think so. We are all sinners! Maybe we don't cheat on our husband, maybe we only abuse him with our angry and hateful words. In my book, the woman who constantly abuses and berates her husband over his past is sinning! She is hurting the marriage tremendously! She is no better than her husband.

God doesn't have different levels of penitence for different sins. A sin is a sin no matter what that sin is. That is why Jesus said to the crowd, "Those WITHOUT SIN cast the first stone." No one could cast a stone at the adulterous woman because they have all sinned! Jesus knew the woman was truly remorseful for what she had done, and that is why he said, "Go and sin no more."

Jesus didn't say, "Those who have not committed adultery cast the first stone." Jesus was telling us how we're all sinners and a sin is a sin in the eyes of God.

"Woman where are they? Has no one condemned you?"
"No one sir, " she said.
"Then neither do I condemn you," Jesus declared. "Go and leave your life of sin."

This is how we are supposed to forgive our husband. Can we cast a stone at our husband?

So what else can a wife do to forgive her cheating husband?

1. She needs to come out of her selfishness and forgive her husband with completeness of her heart and stop dwelling on what was and start fixing what is!

True forgiveness means a change of heart. If we say that we have forgiven but in our heart we are still bitter and angry then we have not "really" forgiven but "really" lied to our self.

Scripture reveals, "The good man brings good things out of the good stored up in his heart, and the evil man brings evil things out of the evil stored up in his heart. For out of the overflow of his heart his mouth speaks." Luke 6:45

True forgiveness only comes from having Faith in Jesus Christ. Why is that? Because it is through Christ that WE HAVE BEEN FORGIVEN. Take Jesus Christ out of the equation, God forbid, and forgiveness of our sins would be no more! With God's help we can accept Christ's forgiveness and stop in our wrongdoing. Scripture tells us that, "God made him who had no sin to be sin for us, so that in him we might become the righteousness of God." 2 Corinthians 5:21

This scripture is talking about a simple exchange and it works like this, our sins were given over to Jesus Christ at His crucifixion and His righteousness is given to us when we believe. Without belief or acceptance in the source of true forgiveness we will be unable to forgive others when they sin against us. ♥

Heal Marriage After Adultery
7

Do you want your marriage nursed back to health? If you want your marriage restored it will take some effort on your part. Stop seeking help from the standards of society and start looking for truth from the source of who you are. God's foundation for marriage is the source for healing your marriage from the tribulations of unfaithfulness in marriage.

First of all I'm hoping that you have decided to forgive completely, and secondly, your husband needs to understand why he strayed from the marriage bed in the first place. The issue of unfaithfulness needs both husband and wife involved within its structure for the marriage to be restored.

Understand that Infidelity is only a symptom of a greater problem within the framework of the marriage. If your husband has been unfaithful and he is repentant of his weakness he needs to find out why he might have been disloyal. He must not blame you for his actions either, this is wrong. Your husband needs to grow up and take responsibility for his actions. He is responsible for his actions and is accountable for those actions to God and to you.

I marvel at how often I hear couples blame each other for being unfaithful. Actually it is a problem within the adulterer themselves that is the root to unfaithfulness. Husbands and wives need to be looking for ways they can please each other instead of bringing each other down into their weakness.

If you're ready to start trusting your husband again and start loving him freely with no conditions to be met, then it is time to tell him so. It takes willingness and effort to seek out everything that God wants for you and your marriage. It is God's will that you continue working on establishing for your marriage a foundation based on trust, respect, commitment and honor. Without these traits imbedded into your belief system, you will have a difficult time trusting your husband. Forgiveness always comes with time; time to see for yourself that your husband loves you and is willing to give up his erring ways and work on the marriage with you.

If your husband is willing to give up his sinful weakness and truly wants to do what is right for the marriage, God has already forgiven him! Knowing this, that is what you both can work off of to help restore it. Through His death, Jesus Christ has paid the price to release your husband from the bondage of sinful immorality.

As his wife, can you accept that? Can you accept that your husband has been forgiven on the basis of the suffering and physical death of Jesus Christ? Acceptance of this great truth and your own willingness to forgive your husband of unfaithfulness will begin the new foundation for your marriage. If you answered yes, then you can rely on Jesus Christ for your new way of living and know that it is God's will for you.

We all have heard about the woman in the Bible caught in the act of adultery. This is how much forgiveness and love we have from God and what Jesus said on that subject.

"The teachers of the law and the Pharisees brought in a woman caught in adultery. They made her stand before the group and said to Jesus, "Teacher, this woman was caught in the act of adultery. In the law, Moses commanded us to stone such a woman. Now what do you say?"

"If any one of you is without sin, let him be the first to throw a stone at her."

At this, those who heard began to go away one at a time, the older ones first, until only Jesus was left, with the woman still standing there. Jesus straightened up and asked her, "woman, where are they? Has no one condemned you?"

"No one, sir," she said.

"Then neither do I condemn you," Jesus declared. "Go now and leave your life of sin." John 8:3:11

What a beautiful scripture on what true forgiveness is. You can support your marriage on the Divine Truth of the realization that your sins are forgiven, start over anew and embrace all that you have been blessed with in your present situation and hold on to what you have. Be willing to reestablish the bonds of trust and respect for each other. Base your love and actions upon the spirit of Jesus Christ. Center your communication with one another around Gods word by taking the time to study and search scripture.

Marriage is tough! There is no disagreement there. The ability to accept, forgive and love must be honored and cherished everyday. You need to honor and respect your husband and he needs to honor and respect you. You cannot tell him to respect you. That won't work. You need to do it first and then he will do the same. We really need to accept our husband as the head of the home, and try and stop analyzing, reviewing, and basing the marriage upon our husband's faults and weakness.

Did you know that with God's guidance we can learn to humble our proud and selfish ego? We will see beyond the faults of our husband and learn to forgive him with the loving kindness, that if he is remorseful for his actions, he deserves from us.

A marriage is only as strong as its foundation. The groundwork for all marriage is adopting the Spirit of Jesus Christ and inviting Him into our lives. He is the support, which holds up the marriage when under pressure.

Scripture reveals in 1 Corinthians 3:11 "For no one can lay any foundation other than the one already laid, which is Jesus Christ."

I believe the seven aspects I have outlined below are the first steps towards rebuilding trust for your marriage.

1.) You will need to forgive with completeness to reestablish the bond you once had with your husband, and bring the relationship to its full potential.

2.) Husband needs to cease in his unfaithfulness

3.) Communicate effectively with your husband through the use of expressing his positive attributes, and talking out your thoughts and feelings with care.

4.) Acceptance of your husband's faults must be established. We all have faults; quit looking at his all the time, and start recognizing some of your own.

5.) Study scripture together for knowledge, truth, and wisdom that your marriage needs most. This gives you both the notice of your commitment in the marriage and boosts the willingness to try even harder.

6.) Time will tell. Experiencing the rightful actions of your husband will eventually bring back the trust that was tampered with.

7.) Roles, positions and responsibilities of both of you need to be honored and respected. Couples need to place more value and importance on their responsibilities by reassuring one another from time to time.

Now you can see from the seven attributes above, you only need to put forth a little bit of spiritual effort. What's wrong with that? Your marriage won't be nursed back to health overnight, but by showing each other the willingness to trust God and to put Him first in your own life does show your husband what your true intentions are for the marriage. Show your man you love him. ♥

Detach With Love
8

As we all know there are times in marriage when we need to detach from the man we married. How do we do that without offending or hurting him? How about with a little bit of compassion and love? It is far better to detach with love then to burst out with angry, destructive, or negative feelings. When we detach it gives us some time to think about the situation at length and then come back to our husband with a satisfying solution.

What happens when we don't detach? Often times we come on too harsh with our feelings. We don't think before we spew out emotional garbage out at our husband. Feelings are great for expressing ourselves but if we use destructive feelings to abuse or otherwise keep us from finding a solution to our marital issues then feelings become a problem.

If we use impulsive and reckless feelings to dictate how we will treat our husband it can become the way we decide to deal with all marital issues until it becomes a habitual way of behaving. If we let our feelings determine how we will love, we certainly won't be able to deal with issues appropriately. Unfortunately, many marriages are like this; couples literally feed off of the feelings of each other. But in reality destructive feelings starve the marriage of nutrients.

For instance, your husband's reaction to your reaction might trigger off a certain set of thoughtless feelings that he has been played out before, but the issue never gets resolved, therefore the root of the problem gets put on the backburner with all the rest of the garbage that didn't get fed properly. As you can easily see it takes spiritual effort on both sides to have an almost idyllic marriage we read about in storybooks. It takes spiritual effort to stay married! Instead of looking for reasons to leave the marriage, we can learn to detach with love, which takes the spiritual resolve that I am talking about.

There is a difference between just detaching from our spouse and detaching WITH LOVE. Detaching with angry feelings and not caring about our spouse is detaching inappropriately. This is not the kind of detachment I'm talking about. Detaching with love is considering our spouses feelings and accepting who they are. Sometimes it is just better to give up and give in rather than get in a messy and heated argument that isn't going anywhere anyway. It is at these times we can detach from our partner with love. When we detach in this way we come away feeling better emotionally and spiritually. And that is what we're looking for here, to *feel* better emotionally and spiritually.

Detaching with love means to turn the other cheek. For instance if your husband is not doing anything hostile to you or the marriage, but is behaving antagonistic for the heck of it, often times turning the other cheek is the better way to go. Detaching in this way becomes a learned way of behavior, which is far better for your psyche and far better for your husbands psyche as well. As difficult as it may seem to do, learning to be more accepting, caring and loving, and just letting *it* go is detaching with the love that I am talking about. When you humble yourself and turn the other cheek you will feel so much better about yourself and about your husband. Being humble and kind is not as hard as it seems, especially when we see for ourselves the positive results it brings into the marriage!

Detaching with love is being humble, forgiving, and accepting. Demonstrating all of these wonderful character traits is being loving towards the man you married. On the other side of the coin, while in a heated battle with your husband, angry words will inhibit all of those traits from your mind and the angry words end up controlling your behavior. Is that what you want? Is that who you are?

Remember, take it one day at a time, and don't look at it as if you have to carry around those character traits twentyfour-seven. No one is perfect. But just knowing when you might be using destructive feelings when dealing with marital issues is a big start to being humble and kind through proper expression of yourself.

Scripture says, "Be completely humble and gentle; be patient, bearing with one another in love. Make every effort to keep the unity of the Spirit through the bond of peace." Ephesians 4:2-3

No marriage is ever perfect here on earth; it just isn't going to happen. But we can certainly enjoy the husband we are married to by putting forth a little bit more effort. We must learn to accept our man and love him in spite of his faults if we want to be satisfied in our marriage. When we see faults in our husband that seem to drive us nuts, instead of harping on him about them, we ought to try and be gentle, kind, and patient like scripture above says.

Does your husband's actions or personality sometimes annoy you? Rather then dwelling on your husband's weakness or looking for faults, detach with love.

When you continue being kind, gentle and loving, you will see that you will want to spend more time with your husband because you have LEARNED to accept him for who he is, faults and all. ♥

5 Biblical Facts About Temptation
9

What is temptation really all about? Satan tempted Eve in the Garden of Eden, and Jesus in the desert. Guess what? Satan tempts you and I every day too. Satan is nothing but a fallen angel gone bad. Satan is an evil spirit who disguises him self to us in deceiving ways. He tempts us into doing immoral things that make us want to live his way instead of God's way, but marriage cannot take this kind of deceit, it will not flourish with Satan being its leader.

1.) Satan likes to tempt people when they are at their most vulnerable, or when they are physically and emotionally overstressed.

"Then Jesus was led by the Spirit into the desert to be tempted by the devil. After fasting forty days and forty nights, he was hungry. The tempter came to him and said, "If you are the Son of God, tell these stones to become bread."
Jesus answered, "It is written: Man does not live on bread alone, but from every word that comes from the mouth of God." Matthew 4:2-4

Satan tempted Jesus after fasting for forty days, and He was hungry and tired. This time of testing showed that Jesus really was the Son of God, because he overcame the temptations of the devil.

God will test all Christian's sometime in their lives. Our convictions are only strong if they will hold up under the pressures of temptation. Are you ready to be tested by Satan?

2.) Satan offered Jesus the whole world because he wanted Jesus to obey him.

Again, the devil took him to a very high mountain and showed him all the kingdoms of the world in their splendor.

"All this I will give you," he said, "if you will bow down and worship me."

Jesus said to him, "Away from me Satan! For it is written: Worship the Lord your God, and serve him only." Matthew 4:8-11

Satan tempts you and I today in the same way by enticing us through the love of money, and power in the world, and by our greed, desire and wants. What temptations have enticed you?

3.) Sin comes in alluring and persuasive forms.

"If you are the Son of God, "he said, "Throw yourself down. For it is written: "He will command his angels concerning you, and they will lift you up in their hands, so that you will not strike a foot against a stone."

Jesus answered him and said, "It is also written, "Do not put the Lord your God to the test." Matthew 4:6-7

Satan used scripture to try and get Jesus to do what he wanted, but Jesus did not falter. Satan made it sound so persuasive, and still Jesus did not sin! When we are tempted, Satan will focus on three areas that he knows we are at our most vulnerable.

1.) Wants, desires (physical) having sex before marriage, immoral and lustful acts, adultery, prostitution, homosexuality, perverted acts, etc.

2.) Materialism, money, power (mental) greed, striving for more money and power makes us not want to get to know God. Striving for status in life makes us rebellious to the ways of God.

3.) Pride! Did you know that our pride is what stands in the way of becoming humble? This is why we are tempted. Pride is the root of number two! Pride is being selfish and rebellious to others. Pride shows up in our feelings and attitude in life. What is your attitude like?

Have you ever been persuaded or convinced to sin? How has Satan persuaded you? Here is what one single young girl wrote to me about regarding her addiction to psychics.

…. Then, my addiction came about--I started calling Psychics... There were many times that they have predicted things to unfold very accurately that I was amazed, and I became a regular caller in regards to my relationships--how he may be thinking, feeling, how he will act, what will happen, will he come around, etc? I am very ashamed about this and have tried to stop myself from calling for several months but eventually repeat the same habit. I've lost so much money on this as well. I logically know that this is very foolish thing to do as an intellectual person who has gained many people's respect in what I do and, overall, as a Christian, who also has participated in missions.

After reading your January newsletter issue on Spiritual life as a Christian, I have decided to email you, with my unresolved issue. I've started Q.T every night, reading His Word, and praying to God... Yet, I am just so tired of my heartaches over the failed relationships and my stupidity in this addiction of Psychic callings. Would you pray for me??? Would you have any advice for me? Exhausted, help!

I did have advice for this young girl. I believe Satan was tempting her to call on psychics instead of on God. Hopefully she will become more spiritually aware before she gets married and calls on fortunetellers for her marital problems as well. We must seek the truth for our answers from a biblical standpoint. Here is what I explained to this young girl.

Fortunetellers and psychics are false interpretations of what is truth and wisdom. Fortunetellers know their job well and that is why many things seem to be accurate, but it is an illusion to keep you coming back for more. I know it is tempting to continue hearing what you want to hear and that is how Satan gets you to keep coming back to psychics for your answers instead of from God where the real answers are.

What is true is already in your heart...you said that you know it is foolish...and so there lies your answer. The Spirit within you (Holy Spirit of Jesus Christ) has given you the answer. Put your faith in God and the temptation and addiction to call on fortunetellers will go away from you.

Don't give up hope on finding the right person for you in your life. You are still young—don't be in such a hurry. Wait on Him for His will and purpose for you. God is with you every step of the way. We here at Heaven Ministries are praying for you. In Christ's love, peace, hope and happiness.

4. God will never lead us into temptation, but He will test us.

..."And Lead us not into temptation, but deliver us from the evil one." Matthew 6:13

All Christians struggle with temptations. Sometimes these tempting situations are so subtle that we don't even know we are sinning. But God has *promised* us that we won't be tempted beyond what we can bear.

Here is a beautiful example of a happily married woman. I am glad that she knows it! It is these kinds of emails I enjoy getting from my readers.

You wrote and excellent article about God's design for marriage. I just want you to know how truly blessed I am to be an adopted child of the Most High God and to have a Beautiful Christian Marriage.

All married women can feel blessed and loved like in their marriage. This Christian woman obviously searched scripture, found her answers and put her faith and trust in God.

It just takes a bit of spiritual awareness to attain a blessed filled marriage. You already have the spirit within you; now all you have to do is learn to use it for the good in your marriage by applying it into the marriage on an everyday basis until it becomes a habit.

"No temptation has seized you except what is common to man. And God is faithful; he will not let you be tempted beyond what you can bear. But when you are tempted, he will also provide a way out so that you can stand up under it." 1 Corinthians 10:13

    4.) Married couples can resist temptations of sexual sin.

    God gives married couples the strength and desire to want to overcome sexual sin. Married couples only need to take their marriage back to the biblical standpoints where it belongs. This will give couples the commitment their marriage deserves and sexual sin would be eliminated all together.

"The husband should fulfill his marital duty to his wife, and likewise the wife to the husband. The wife's body does not belong to her alone but also to her husband. In the same way, the husband's body does not belong to him alone, but also to his wife. Do not deprive each other except by mutual consent

and for a time, so that you may devote yourselves to prayer.
Then come together again so Satan will not tempt you
because of your lack of self-control." 1 Corinthians 7:3-5

Spiritually we belong to God, but physically we belong to our
spouse! ❤

5 Biblical Aspects On Forgiveness
10

I talk a lot about forgiveness in marriage and relationships. Why? Because without forgiving those who have wronged us, we will never be able to forget the wrong either. And when I say, "forget", I mean in the sense that the wrong will never be brought up again to hurt or otherwise abuse our spouse with.

I have outlined five biblical aspects on learning to forgive properly.

1. Forgiveness is the first step in repairing/restoring relationships.

The bible reveals to us, "But I tell you that anyone who divorces his wife, except for marital unfaithfulness, causes her to become an adulteress, and anyone who marries the divorced woman commits adultery. Matthew 5:32

Divorce is hurtful and destructive and God intends for marriage to be a lifetime commitment. Genesis 2:24.

This is precisely why couples should never consider divorce an option for solving marital problems, and here's why. Jesus said that divorce was not permissible except for unfaithfulness, but...this does not mean, and is not saying that a spouse should automatically get a divorce because a spouse commits adultery!

The word translated "unfaithfulness" means LIVING in a sexually immoral lifestyle, not a repented act of adultery. There is a BIG difference here between a continual lifestyle of sexual sin and a one-time affair.

Those women who have found their husbands to be unfaithful should make every effort to forgive and restore their marriage.

2. God does not forgive those who do not forgive others

The bible tell us again, "For if you forgive men when they sin against you, your heavenly Father will also forgive you. But if you do not forgive men their sins, your Father will not forgive your sins." Matthew 6: 14-15

The simple truth is when we don't forgive others we are denying our common ground as sinners in need of God's forgiveness. We all need to be forgiven at times, and we are all sinners! When we ask for forgiveness from God and others, we should ask ourselves, "Have I forgiven the people who have wronged me?"

It is all about putting our selves in their shoes. We can't honestly expect to be forgiven when we can't seem to forgive others! We all need forgiven and we all must forgive! It's really that simple.

Do you need to forgive your husband? Does your husband need to forgive you? Submit to one another through forgiveness and restore the trust and respect that may have been misplaced. Forgiving others takes humbleness, no doubt about it, and humbling ourselves is difficult to do, especially if we are angry or hurt. But it is absolutely what we must do to be able to forgive properly!

I receive a flood of emails and letters from couples about how to forgive their spouse. Here is one that fits in with what this chapter is saying.

I am struggling with every relationship because I have a hard time forgiving people who have done me wrong. I do want to forgive but because I have a hard time forgetting the incidents, I have a hard time letting go of the past. People do not understand me, and why I cannot forgive them sooner.... I am fasting today so God can intervene in my life so that I may not struggle in this particular area anymore. I need some time off and cool down before returning to the person when I am ready to talk about my emotions objectively. But most of the times most people are not very patient with me. I was wondering if this is a biblical way of resolving differences. This is the only way I know how to resolve differences with people. And some people are pressuring me to change so drastically. I feel so unwelcome and unloved by this particular crowd.

Do you have any word of advice? Please be in prayer for me.

Yes, I did have a lot of advise for this person. The first and foremost important piece of advice that I gave her was to read and study the bible for more spiritual awareness. Start by going to the concordance and looking up the word "forgive" and follow it to the scriptures.

She talks a lot about how others have wronged her. Well has she stopped to think that maybe she has wronged them too? No, she probably hasn't done that because she isn't aware that she has wronged anyone, it's all about her. So my next word of advice for her, and I know it sounds strong, was for her to come out of her selfishness, humble her self to the living God, and learn to understand who *she is,* and then, she won't feel like the victim anymore.

If we feel like victims all the time then we will not be able to truly forgive. Feeling like the victim keeps us living inside of our resentment and at times can manifest into "the world owes me a favor" kind of attitude. Unfortunately, this woman has some negative emotions that need healed, and only God

58

can heal those feelings for her.

Thirdly, I commended her on her willingness to "cool off" first before she confronted the person she needed to forgive. Lots of times after we have thought about the incident and the hurt, we realize that we can forgive properly. Lastly I explained to her that maybe she should reexamine the crowd of people she is hanging around with. I was prompted to tell her to have discernment in the friends she chooses because many times friends are not friends at all but our enemies. Why would she feel so unloved and unwanted around friends?

3. True forgiveness is found only from having faith in Jesus Christ

True forgiveness is found only from having faith in Jesus? Really?

Jesus says, "If you forgive anyone his sins, they are forgiven; if you do not forgive them, they are not forgiven." John 20:23

It's as simple as that?

In the above scripture Jesus was giving the disciples their Spirit-powered and Spirit-guided mission, which was to teach the good news about Jesus so people's sins would and could be forgiven.

But the disciples did not have the power to forgive sins, but Jesus gave them the opportunity of telling new believers that their sins have been forgiven because they had ACCEPTED Jesus' message. Because of their belief in Jesus, they were given the power within them to FORGIVE!

All believers have this same opportunity today! We can announce the forgiveness of sins with certainty when we ourselves have found repentance and faith in Christ. Wow!

4. Forgiveness will lead to a change of heart

Isn't this great news! Jesus is simply saying that he will forgive us when we have faith enough in him to turn our life around and sin no more. This is true forgiveness.

When Jesus said that only a sinless person could throw the first stone at the adulterous woman, he was actually highlighting several important areas in our own lives that we need to watch out for, such as forgiving others, showing compassion, and not to judge others who have sinned.

5. Forgiveness involves both attitude and action on our part

The Bible says, "Do not take revenge, my friends, but leave room for God's wrath, for it is written" "It is mine to avenge' I will repay, says the Lord. On the contrary: "if your enemy is hungry, feed him' if he is thirsty, give him something to drink. In doing this, you will be heap burning coals upon his head." Romans 12:19-21

By giving an enemy a drink, we are not excusing his misdeeds, but forgiving him and loving him despite of his sins. Jesus Christ did this for us. This is called "detaching with love", or Jesus called it, "turning the other cheek."

Forgiveness does involve a good attitude on our part. Many times we find it too difficult to forgive. We just don't feel very forgiving towards someone who has hurt us. It is at these times that we must try to be kind towards him or her. Being kind to people who have hurt us tends to ease the hurt and makes us feel better towards them in our heart and mind.

Sometimes we need to do things we don't want to. But we'll soon discover that by doing kind things to those who have hurt us can actually lead to our feelings changing for the good. We can love our husbands. ❤

My Husband Looks At Pornography - Is That The Same As Adultery?
11

Computers can be used for the good, but they can also be used for corruption. We have choices we can look, or we can choose not to look.

Pornography has snuck into our homes like Satan did with Eve in the Garden of Eden, tempting even the purest of heart. Some people have never thought about looking at porn before they had a computer, but now it somehow repeatedly gets in their view, and oops it happens.

There are a few really bad apples out there that revel and delight in tossing immoral imagery into our faces. Whether we read about these lusty desires in our Spam email or see it on popup banners, we've all come face to face with it through our computer. Most of us don't think twice about deleting porn from our email and in fact, we try to get popup blocker to stop the harassing banner ads. Since porn is tossed out recklessly everyday in front of our face, eventually someone is going to click on it. It might be your husband, daughter, or teenage son.

The bad apples are overjoyed! They work for Satan. Satan tells them sneaky and conniving ways how to do it, and make it more enticing. The bad apples comply because they want everyone to be depraved like them.

The problem begins when a person is tempted into viewing this garbage and they do not apply any moral ethics they might have on a godly foundation.

The worldview of what morality is in grave error. If you base your belief system on something that is sinful, you will become in bondage to that particular sin. That is how Satan gets people involved in his work. They serve him by being a slave to sin.

Because porn repeatedly shows up on our computer in one form or another, we eventually give into it out of curiosity and think. *"One time won't hurt"*. In reality, folks, it does hurt. It hurts yourself and your loved ones tremendously.

"You have heard that it was said, "Do not commit adultery. But I tell you anyone who looks at a woman lustfully has already committed adultery with her in his heart."
Matthew 5:27,28

Here is what the Bible says about looking at pornography.

1. Lust is an unhealthy and sinful desire that takes a person away from that which is right and good. It does not matter if it is lusting after strangers on the Internet or a fleshly body in a secret place. To yearn for the flesh of another person other than who you are married is wrong thinking taking over your mind and eliminating the natural goodness that resides in man.

Ladies, if your husband has been looking at pornography, it is time to let him know that you know about it. It is time to properly discuss the issue behind *why* your husband might be looking at pornography. Obviously looking at pornography is a symptom of a greater underlying problem within your husband. Find out what that problem is and fix it.

Satan knows that men like visionary images brought to their mind. Once a man pictures an image in his mind, he continues to see that image for day's sometimes-even weeks. Women forget about it the very same day.

Satan knows that by getting your husband to think, and then envision the lusty images in his mind first will entice him to desire it, more and more. Once your man takes a peek, he is likely to peek again, and again, until he can't seem to get the immoral imagery away from his mind, and he becomes ensnared within it.
This is how addiction gets started. If you think long enough, you become what you think. God says we are not to even THINK about these things in our mind.

"Do not lust in your heart after her beauty or let her captivate you with her eyes, for the prostitute reduces you to a loaf of bread, and the adulteress preys upon your very life". Proverbs 25, 26

Your husband needs to feel special by you. He needs to know that he is worth more than a loaf of bread by you. Pray and study the bible daily together. Take God breathed counsel seriously. Be committed to your marriage and put in extra effort to do whatever it takes to help your husband stop his addiction.

2. If the *act* of adultery is wrong, then so is the *intention*. It is considered mental adultery and thus a sin! To be faithful to your wife with your body, but not your mind is to break the trust that is so vital to marriage.

Pornography is easily justified in the minds of the husband's that view it. They have broken a code of ethics to validate in their minds that it is okay to view it. Pornography for many is more justified than the physical act and if they get caught looking at it, all they have to say is, "Well, at least I didn't have an affair." But this kind of thinking is wrong and is in total denial. Denial is the opposite of acceptance. If your husband can't accept that what he is doing is wrong then he is in denial, plain and simple!

The Internet only enables those who are tempted to continue in their addiction. Satan instructs the bad apples to get smarter and smarter in their different ways to put it out to the world. That means you have to fight back harder to eliminate sexual immorality from your life. Maybe you need to put a filter on your computer, or better yet, maybe you and your husband can turn to God for deliverance from the temptation.

"It is God's will that you should be sanctified: that you should avoid sexual immorality; that each of you should learn to control his own body in a way that is holy and honorable, not in passionate lust like the heathen, who do not know God." 1Thessalonians 4, 3-5

Viewing Pornography and getting off on a temporary rush is only a symptom of a much greater problem. Lusting after the flesh of heathen strangers is bad enough, but this lustful desire also defiles the body, mind, soul, and marriage. In my book, it is the same as having a physical affair.

This does not mean that you cannot forgive this particular sin or that God will not forgive the repentant heart. On the contrary, by forgiving and acknowledging God as your source of forgiveness, it will give each of you a new found freedom to love and accept one another under God's loving foundation. The truth is what sets us free from sin!

How can a man stop looking at pornography? The power to rid him self of temptation and to remain faithful comes from what he believes. Therefore it does not rest in him alone but in God. If your husband has been looking at pornography it is because he doesn't have the foggiest idea how to utilize the tools (gifts) God has given him. God can and will forgive your husband and give him a new heart to lead him.

Understand that loyalty to our spouse is a part of the giving process that we learn by allowing God's love and forgiveness into our heart and mind. We become what we have accepted already from God; we become forgiveness and we become love by our actions. In other words, when we accept God's love for us that is when we can actually give of our self to others and to do it freely. It's really that simple. Accepting is on the same line as humbling oneself. If we humble our self to God, the one and only true director, we are giving our self to God and our spouse. Once we actually release our errors to God, He will rid us of being tempted in our life and marriage.

For those of you who might be reading this and your conscience is kicking you in the face, I say don't kick your self too hard. You made a mistake and looked at porn. Pick yourself right back up and start all over anew. I say the same thing for those individuals who have had an affair. Just because you were weak once does not mean you are a weak person. You are what you believe to be true. Your potential is much greater than you allow. God will give you the power to cease and desist all tempting situations in your life, and become the person you were intended to be. But you have to accept and believe that God's plan is what works, not the worlds.

God hasn't condemned you yet. It is not too late to turn your life around and come to your full potential. Let go of Satan's hand and take a hold of Christ's hand. Don't condemn yourself! Don't forget, God is your source so don't look to the world (Satan) for reassurance of self? If the world is where you look for truth, you will believe what the world says, and probably be weak in your sin again.

Here is what one of the Heaven Ministries newsletter subscribers wrote in and told me. Thankfully, he was ready to look away from his sin and accept Christ in his life.

I have made my wife's life miserable because I have an addiction to porn, at first I did not want to admit it, but I now realize that I have to let it go to save my marriage. My wife has not left me yet...but I know that she is at the point where she wants to go away. I can't live without her and I realize that a slave cannot have two masters...I chose my wife so what can I do to rebuild my marriage? Please help save my marriage.

Fortunately this husband is on the right path. He knows that looking at pornography is wrong and he obviously has a repentant heart. The next step for him is to apply God's goodness into the marriage by giving his sin(s) to God. You do not have to step into a Church to do this. God can hear your cries and suffering wherever you are. Accepting Christ's forgiveness, and having faith and trust in God that he can help you with your weakness will keep the marriage from falling, for you have chosen the righteous foundation to work off of.

As with any addiction we are powerless to defeat it on our own. I know this first hand; I have been there and done that with an addiction to alcohol for many years. When we fall into weakness, essentially, we're like a confused lost puppy unable to find our way home. We do not have a map to help us search for the lost treasure. We're probably not even sure why we are unfaithful and some of us remain in weakness. We might be so wrapped up in our addiction (sin) that we cannot find the right path because we think we're already on the right path. We have decided that society is our home, and society tells us that unfaithfulness is acceptable. Which, on the opposite end is what God says is not acceptable.

As I said earlier, when we accept what we see in the world as truth, we tempt our self into adultery and immorality of all kinds, which is not truth, but a devilish lie told by Satan. We have to come to God and realize that we are powerless without him!

Bottom line: It is God's will that marriage be built upon the rock of loyalty and when a man learns to remain steadfast and loyal to his wife, he will be allowing God to give him the understanding he needs to remain faithful. By trusting in what God says for his marriage, he will be less tempted to stray from the marriage bed, whether in the physical act or through pornography.

If your husband has an addiction to pornography he needs to be willing to stop the addiction and accept Jesus Christ, instead of society for the answers. Faith comes from believing in what we cannot see with our eyes, bringing those beliefs into our heart and acting upon them with passion. Having and utilizing the power of faith is an individual matter that is gained by having a personal relationship with God. You need to make God your source for your marriage!

It is not to late to come out of Sodom & Gomorrah. Your husband can find his way home and you can help him find the doorbell. ♥

Working Faith For My Marriage
12

Every happy and content filled marriage possesses confidence and faith in God. A husband who has faith in the Lord has the faith to lead his family righteously. He has faith enough in God to live by Gods infallible truths for marriage.

A woman whose husband has faith in the Lord has faith enough in her self as a woman to be a respectful wife and loving mother. She has faith enough to submit to her husband's spiritual authority knowing that she is not giving up her identity as a woman but is gaining the wisdom and righteousness of God. Can you see then how couples having faith and trust in God makes for a great marriage?

Faith is derived through complete trust and belief in God. That's all about it. Faith is brought into the marriage by using the power of it through our convictions and beliefs. Faith becomes apparent in our lives when we are constant with our prayer and daily living and through Gods words and Holy Spirit within us.

Though God hears our prayers, they may not get answered the way we think they should. What we want and ask for in our prayers is probably not what God wants for us.

Many of us pray only when we are in dire need of something. But this is not using faith properly. This is being selfish to God.

We can find faith through the understanding of how God works through the Christian's life. We must always seek His will for our lives when praying and through that faith prayers will be answered. When we utilize our faith through the word of Jesus Christ, we are doing the will of God. In other words, if we are lacking in faith it is because we have stopped pursuing God's word because staying faithful is an ongoing matter. Participating in Church services on Sunday is not enough to keep the faith. We must humble ourselves to Him at all times, and in all things, and let Him decide what is best for us.

Romans says, "Consequently, faith comes from hearing the message, and the message is heard through the word of Jesus Christ." Romans 10:17

We also gain more faith by acting on it. When we act on faith because of our belief in God that means we trust in what God says he is going to do for our lives, instead of using self-based faith.

One woman wrote to me feeling discouraged and on the verge of giving up, here is what she said.

My question is how do I keep a marriage alive when I have been separated 10 years as my husband is in Prison in the mainland. He has another 10 years to do. I am in Hawaii and we don't see each other for years on end. No contact. Feel single, can' t remember what marriage is. Kids hurt. I hurt and ache all time from missing him. My flesh is torn. I don't know if I can wait another 10 years. I have prayed and stood and held on for life. My husband keeps telling me to move on. He does not understand how I can wait. Lost all my family and friends nearly over this marriage. Help! Any wisdom would be appreciated.

I told her how important it is to trust in what God says is true and that he will do what he says he'll do according to his word. Faith comes from trusting in God. I told her how her faith would eventually reflect back onto her husband. He will recognize her faith and begin to have faith in God as well. No matter what happens she is still married to that man in prison and if she remarries while he is still alive, she will be committing adultery. He needs to know that also. Instead of looking for ways to leave or get out of the marriage, they should be looking for ways to get closer to God and to each other. Maybe writing letters on a daily basis will keep them close in heart and mind. I know that ten years is a long time to be without the man you love and married, but with God in the picture both of them can find comfort through their love letters, and even become more bonded because of it!

Here is a person who emailed me wanting to know if he can continue sinning even though he has tried to give them up.

There are sins that I love, and I try to give them up but I just can't do it. Will God count me as an enemy even though I try and fail? Will he send me to hell even though I am sorry for my sins, but I keep going back to them?

I told him how important it is for him to be reading and studying the Bible on a daily basis, even if it is only three or four verses at a time. It is what will bring him closer to the Lord and help him to stop sinning. Studying the bible is what gives us more faith. Praying daily is what will help us to question our motives about sin. It doesn't happen in a day or even a month, it is a continual process of learning and growing, and accepting Christ for our lives instead of the sin we are relying on now. Once we accept Christ, we won't need the sin in our lives anymore. This is how it works! It just takes more spiritual effort, that's all. We continue to commit the same sin because we haven't asked God to free us from it yet.
     We should never stop praying for what God wants for us

in our marriage. Too many times we pray out of selfishness and ask of God those things which WE WANT. This is why prayers are not answered. We wonder what all this faith stuff is about since our prayers are not being met. But God does not work like this.

Faith is a tool that God gives us because He wants us to use it for our salvation and he has gifted us with the ability to put our complete trust and faith in Him. Trusting in God gives you the faith you need in submitting to your husbands protection and love for you. Love the man you married. ♥

How to be More Assertive with Your Husband
13

Anyone can be assertive but it involves practice. We can't just one day say, "Hey I'm going to be assertive today." We have to realize the times when we need to be assertive and practice it. In marriage there are many times when we need to be assertive with our husband. We may need to let them know how we FEEL for instance. Being assertive is good for marriage. I'll tell you why.

1. It lets our husband know how we feel
2. It tells our husband that we have self confidence in what we do
3. It allows us to have what we need and want
4. We become more self assured in everything we do

Assertiveness isn't being aggressive, rude or violent. Assertiveness is expressing our self properly by telling our husband what we want and who we are. I'm going to show you how to be assertive with your husband without being overbearing and aggressive. We don't want to get overbearing, but we do want them to know how we are feeling.

People-pleasing types have a difficult time being assertive because they won't speak up for themselves. They want their husband and friends to be happy, but later feel resentful and needy because of it. We cannot be happy in marriage if we're ALWAYS trying to make our husband happy! Can we? Besides we shouldn't have to "try" to make anyone happy, it should just be a natural occurrence because we are happy with who we are.

Often times when we apply assertive thinking into our life and marriage we realize how much more content we are with our self and others because we are pleasing our self instead of everyone else. We don't have to carry around the baggage of resentment. Resentment? What's that?

When we are self-assured and know what it is we want and need, we become who it is we are and we show others who we are too. We can still please others and be assertive, so we shouldn't become selfish over it, and only consider our feelings. We need to find balance that brings us, as well as our husband, and anyone else in the home, the happiness we all deserve.

I know that many couples struggle in their marriage and it's because of something a husband did or didn't do. These women are unhappy and on the verge of divorce. But you see, if these women would stop focusing on what their husbands did or didn't do, and start focusing on what THEY can do about it, they would begin to "grow out" from the problems they carry from within into the marriage.

Divorce has now become the easy way out. But this is a selfish and unrealistic way to perceive happiness. Happiness is something that you cannot find through others. To gain it, you must go after it. You cannot sit around hoping your husband will change, so you can be happy. You need to do something about it from your end. That is where assertiveness comes in.

Somehow we expect our husband's to know how we are feeling and expect them to cater to our every need. But this isn't right. We can't expect our husband to know how we're feeling. We need to speak up and tell them, and we can start by being assertive with what we have to say.

If a woman doesn't know "who she is" or what she wants out of life, she will never truly be happy-no matter who she is married to. The grass looks greener on the other side of the fence, but it's a mirage, ladies! We only need to work on making our own lawn lush and green by putting into the marriage a bit more spiritual effort, that's all.

We please our self by being assertive, and when we do assert our self we feel more loving. Love will flow freely from our heart and this is real love. Real love doesn't have any conditions or stipulations that need met, because we have already taken care of what we want for our selves by being assertive! This is the kind of love that we all want, but no one ever seems to get. When we are happy and peaceful with who we are, we certainly don't need to be sponging off our husband for happiness. We can give them more room to be who it is they are too. And now, instead of both spouses' being unhappy and miserable in the marriage, they both can be happy together!

Ironically, the more we please our self, the better wife we become. With our needs fulfilled, we will have so much more to give. Husbands prefer their wives to be assertive with them. They actually want to please their wives. They want their wives to be happy. But all too often husbands don't know what it is their wife needs because she doesn't speak up for her self assertively! She wants to please everyone all the time, but afterwards, she complains about it, but it's too late by then. Sound familiar?

The problem starts when a "people pleaser" wife has given to her limit, and ends up feeling unfulfilled and discontented. Sometimes the need for fulfillment comes in the form of desperation, and causes all sorts of problems in the marriage.

Bang! The grass seems very green on the other side of the fence again. Now what? Couples aren't being assertive enough to tell each other what it is they want. Expectations become so huge that when they aren't fulfilled, disappointment and resentment steps in. But someone in the marriage needs to break this pattern before things get out of hand. Don't expect your husband to do this. Hang-up the pride and start considering the man you married. Choose to love. You can start by being assertive about what you really want.

But what about him and his love for you, you might be thinking? Well, if you feel that you aren't getting the respect or love from your husband that you think you're entitled to, what do you think will happen? That's right, you'll start to cling to him for it, by any means possible. You might complain, nag, yell, scream, clam up, and become resentful. The truth is, the more you cling to your husband for happiness and try and control them through your neediness, the more they will back off from you, and the more desperate you'll become.

This is why I stress so often in my articles and e-books that to find happiness, we *first* need to find it from within our self. We teach others by showing.

To get respect, *first* we need to be respectful, to be loved, we first need to be loving. If we find this too difficult to do, then we back away for a while until it becomes easier for us to do. It is God's will that we respect and honor the man we married. Don't beg for happiness from your husband. Seek peace and contentment through the spiritual self. We all have a spirit that God has given us. This spirit within us is all we need to bring happiness and peace into our lives. That means we need to stop looking to what the culture does for their marriage and seek out what God wants for our marriage.

Scripture tells us in 1 Corinthians 2:12, "We have not received the spirit of the world but the Spirit who is from God, that we may understand what God has freely given us."

By utilizing the Spirit of God for your marriage you will be given the understanding to know everything you need to know to be happy, peaceful, and content filled in your marriage. ♥

7 Biblical Facts About Marriage
14

Marriage is God's design. Genesis 2 18-24

God's created work was not complete until he made the beautiful woman. He could have made her out of the dust of the ground as he made man, but he chose to make her from the man's flesh and bones. Now why do you think that is? Man and woman become one in the union of marriage. It takes two to get married but the marriage is one body in Christ.

A couple's purpose and goals should be one and the same as the two work together to live out their purpose and, attain their dreams and aspirations. All throughout the bible God treats this special relationship of marriage seriously. The goal and purpose for marriage is more than friendship; it is oneness. Meaning the two become one in flesh.

Commitment was made to love and honor one another! Genesis 24:58-60

Marriage was not just for convenience sake, nor was it brought about by the culture. It was instituted by God and has three basic aspects.

♥ The man leaves his parents and, in a public act, promises himself to his wife.

♥ The man and woman are joined together by taking responsibility for each other's welfare, and by loving each other above all others.

♥ The two become one flesh in the intimacy and commitment of the sexual union that is reserved for marriage. Strong marriages include all three of these aspects.

Marriage was intended to be permanent!
Matthew 19:6

"So they are no longer two, but one. Therefore what God has joined together, let man not separate."

Jesus focused on marriage rather than divorce.

He pointed out that God intended marriage to be permanent and gave four reasons for the importance of marriage.

1.) God made them male and female,
2.) Man leaves his father and mother and is united to his wife;
3.) The two become one flesh,
4.) What God has joined together let man not separate.

God designed marriage to be indissoluble. Instead of looking for reasons to break it off, we should be trying to find reasons to stay married!

Only death should dissolve marriage! Romans 7:2,3

"For example, by law a woman is bound to her husband as long as he is alive, but if her husband dies, she is released from the law of marriage. So then if she married another man while her husband is still alive, she is called an adulteress."

Marriage is good and honorable Hebrews 13:4

"Marriage should be honored by all, and the marriage bed kept pure, for God will judge the adulterer and all the sexually immoral."

Romance in marriage keeps us from being tempted.

It is important to look for ways to bring romance into your marriage. Song of Songs 4:9,10

> Romance keeps marriage exciting. Commitment keeps romance from diminishing away. The most important decision a woman ever makes in her life is at the altar when she commits her self to her husband for the rest of her life. ♥

How to Not Change Your Husband
15

There has always been a lot of talk about how to change the person we married. Could it be that we actually believe that to be happy we need to change our husband? But we married him! It's absurd to think that our unhappiness has something to do with the man we married. Yes, it is true that when we have a not so good marriage we are unhappy but it takes two to participate in the marriage dance.

Why are we looking to our husband for happiness? It is up to us to make ourselves happy, not the man we married.

The thinking on this particular subject is so out of whack that I decided to turn the tables and write the reasons why we should not change our spouse.

For one thing, loving our husband is giving him the freedom to be who it is he is. When we love without wanting anything in return is when we have accepted our husband for being who he is, faults and all. How can we be loving when we don't like something about the man we married, and we're always trying to change him?

This of course, doesn't include iniquitous behavior because if any husband is carrying on and regularly doing things in err

80

against his wife or God then they certainly are not being the man they were meant to be. Therefore, this point I'm trying to make does not apply here.

God grant me the serenity to accept the things I cannot change! Love is an option; we select the degree of love and what kind of love we will give to our husband through our actions. Love can sometimes be confusing and misleading, especially if couples are going through trials and tribulations in their marriage and are demanding of one another.

We think that if we could change our husband, we'll suddenly be happy and contented with ourselves. I know this because I tried changing my husband for years. We try and change our husband because we have stopped accepting him for who he is. Therefore, we cannot seem to love him either. Pretty soon, we begin to place nasty conditions on the love we give to him. If our husband's faults irritate us bad enough we might not give any love at all. Sound familiar? With no love left to give to our husband, we might think we have nothing in common anymore? Who knows, maybe we begin to think we married the wrong man? Suppose the person we met last week at work is better than our husband? Pretty soon we have brainwashed our self into believing our feelings. We have ultimately controlled a situation because of how we *felt* and made things worse.

No wonder more than half of all marriages end in divorce! How about, God grant me the serenity to accept the things I cannot change! Couples waste so much of their time and energy trying to change each other. But is that really going to work? Marriage gurus think they have all the answers, and self help books goat and challenge couples to try and change for each other. But most of these people are divorced too! So what gives? How a bout a little bit of acceptance! It works wonders.

Really, we just need to try and not let those little things bother us. Even some of the bigger things we can detach from. Forgive. Turn the other cheek. Do these things even when you don't want to! Communicate the issue. Let your husband know what bothers you, but don't make it into a tirade. Don't scream and yell at him about how bad he is, instead find something positive to say about him. Make him feel good about who he is, and then express your feelings. That's what works!!

What about, "I'll scratch your back, if you scratch mine". This is good in marriage. There is nothing wrong with the "give and take" type rapport with each other. In fact, this is essentially how couples love each other. No one can ever love unconditionally, without demands, bargains or expectations, never. You know why? Because we're just human, we err, and we have faults. We need to accept that and move on with our life; hopefully that moving on includes our husband. The "give and take" process is a natural occurrence; it is instinctive to do something nice for our husband because they have done something nice for us. We play the give and take game virtually all day long with most of our interactions in our daily affairs; it's part of life. Most marriages work in this fashion; it is a good way for marriage to flourish and grow. It keeps couples on their toes as far as remembering to "give" of themselves periodically to their spouse even when they don't feel like it. That is love.

Now, there is a big difference when we put ultimatums on the table. Dishing out ultimatums is more of a "nasty conditional love" and is based on selfish thinking and usually stems from a wife harboring resentment. "I'll love you, only if you will stop going out with your friends, etc." This is not love, but a selfish and controlling woman trying to get her way through manipulation and ultimatums!

The truth is most marriages can be salvaged. We have to stop *thinking* we can change our husband. We really just need to try a little bit harder by letting those things go that we can't do anything about, and stop feeling resentful can make a big impact on the marriage.

Ladies, we need to start allowing our husband the freedom to just BE. Accept the man we married and love! Love is created by a person and not just is. Love takes action to accomplish. The value of the love we give to our husband is based on how we are feeling at any given moment and time. Suppose we are feeling bitter and resentful towards our husband for something he did or didn't do, we'll inevitably love with that resentment and bitterness, which is one way we place nasty conditions when we love our man. It happens all the time.

"What is generated from our heart comes out in our actions". Loving someone in the real sense of the word is allowing him or her to be who it is they are. When we learn to play the "give and take" game fairly is when can accept the man we are married to.

Bottom line, accept your husband for who he is, give in to your husband without wanting anything in return, and it will eventually be given back to you. This is how to not change your husband. Acceptance is love. ♥

Communicate Effectively
With Your Husband
16

The art of effective communication is an act of being a good listener and understanding what your husband is trying to say. Communication is a useful tool not only in marriage but also in speech and in writing, for conveying information to others in everyday transactions.

Any woman can become a skilled communicator and effectively interact with her husband. For most women, it's probably easier to be the talker than the listener. But we should try to really listen to what our husband's are saying or at least trying to say, and if we are at all confused at what we are hearing, we need to ask questions!

We're not silly or ignorant because we don't fully understand what our husbands are saying; we just need to ask more questions. We're acting silly when we think we already know what they are saying and take our husbands way of thinking and feelings under our own understanding and dissect it into what we want and think it to be. We certainly don't want to be misinformed, do we? So lets try and understand our husband better.

Some women just aren't that good at expressing their feelings and thoughts the way they really feel because they're afraid of being invalidated by their husbands. But if we don't express ourselves and how we feel properly our man will not see us for whom we really are. When we interact with our husbands through faulty communication it could be detrimental to the relationship and cause all kinds of confusion. Expressing our self with anger in the marriage can cause our husband to feel like we don't love or care about them. It can be very confusing to the man who is taking this abuse. When we act out aggression in a negative way, our husband doesn't understand what we are trying to convey to them, whether it be a complaint or harbored resentment. It's okay to express angry feelings, but to do it in a way that is going to actually assist both of you in getting the issue resolved. Accusing and finger pointing doesn't get feelings and thoughts out appropriately. What does is directing hurt emotions at yourself, instead of at the man you married.

Do say, *"I feel so angry that you spent our vacation money. We both worked hard at saving those funds."*

Don't say, *"You stupid idiot, what is wrong with you, can't you do anything right?"*

Always try to turn the conversation towards self by using phrases like, "I thought," "I feel," "I think," Try not to use finger pointing accusations. This will shut down your husband, and he will scamper away from you.

When dealing with issues within the marriage, I have found that some of us women tend to over-react and go on and on and not really get to the point of what's bothering us. When there is a problem that needs discussed, we may bring up past issues, instead of the issue at hand because we feel resentful. It's hard for anyone to understand this kind of behavior and it feels like we are being nagged at instead of talked to. This is why some of us avoid issues and confrontations or walk away when the heat kicks up. No one wants to be nagged at or put down. Lack of proper

85

communication never solves the problem. More resentment builds up and walking away and ignoring the issue sounds better and better. But we don't want this. That is why we need to learn to react in beneficial ways when our husband upsets us.

Even though we all know that men nag too, we also know that men usually only say their complaint once and that's the end of it. We woman on the other hand seem to keep on nagging, and for good reason, our men aren't hearing us! But why are they not hearing us? Maybe it's because we have a naggy tone and awful attitude about our beef. Have you ever tried whispering? It works!

Our men don't want to be nagged at; they want to be talked to just like we women do. Yelling, nagging, and or behaving nasty will not work. What will is a soft toned voice with a sweet smile. And when trouble does arise in the marriage, and you have a complaint, essentially, husbands need their wives to come right out with what is bothering them when it happens. Don't wait until the moon is full again. He will have forgotten about the issue by then.

For instance, wives, lets say you need your husband to go to the store after he gets off work. You should say something like this, *"John, please go to the grocery store after work, I need bread and milk.* Be assertive in your speech but also be nice and kind.

Don't say, "John, I'm out of bread and milk and I'm really tired tonight. If you have time after work, if you could, please go to the grocery store. But, if you don't want to, I guess that I can just go in the morning."

If you ask in a round-about way, like you don't care if he goes to the store or not, he'll probably not think it very important to go to the store and buy bread and milk and won't go to the store. He heard you say, *if you could,* and or *have time,* thereby thinking the grocery errand to not be very important. Because he didn't go to the grocery store for you, you are now feeling resentful towards him. So the bottom line is, just come right out with what you have to say or what you want with a nice tone in your voice-and it works!

As we know, men on the other hand, when expressing themselves have a tendency to shorten things too much and actually believe their wives can read their minds, which of course, isn't true. We need to tell our husbands that if they are talking to us about something important, it helps to explain in detail what it is they need us to do, because we women need and appreciate more detail. Specify who, what, when, and where and most women will be happy.

For instance, lets say your husband wrote you a note before you left for work asking you to drop the hand truck off at Bill's house. Yet, you and your husband know three different people named Bill, and you're not sure which Bill to give the hand truck to. You call your husband at work but he is in a meeting all day and can't come to the phone. You couldn't get a hold of your husband and so were unable to drop the hand truck off at 'Bill's, even though he promised it to him. You broke your promise to Bill because your husband didn't convey proper detail in his note to you.

So in a nutshell, ladies, we can't read our husband's mind, can we? Let's tell them so because they need to know. We wives need to cut to the chase with our husbands and tell them what it is we really need and want, instead of beating around the bush. Be more assertive in your communication and do it with a smile.

It is so true that men and woman are so different in the way they communicate, but that is precisely why we need to help each other out by being considerate of the fact the men are from Mars and women from Venus.

Good talkers are usually good listeners. And good listeners will speak what they mean. They explain things in such a way that the other person understands exactly what it is they are trying to convey. Expressing thoughts and feelings can be hard to do. Especially when we aren't sure what those thoughts are. We should strive to know what it is we want ourselves before saying something that could invariably bring

on distorted thinking and hearing. Here is what one reader
had to say.

*I must tell you that I just loved the article you wrote on communication
and, could not stop from reading!! I have always been interested in people
relationships (who isn't????), and this article really helped me to solidify
certain beliefs that I kept inside but could not easily manifest in reality
due to a lack of courage. I realize now that in communicating my feelings
in a calm manner with others in times of frustration can really resolve my
stress that I have been experiencing lately these days. It will actually
make my life easier. Of course, the unconditional love I would require to
carry out the communication in the right way so that it will not result in
arguments. Only thing that really worries me is does this unconditional
love thing really apply to dating relationships? Should I let the man I'm
with know how I really feel...wouldn't this usually sabotage the
development of the relationship that it may "scare off" the man?*

She is right in being calm when communicating herself. As
we all know, communication backed by anger never gets the
reaction we are looking for. In response to this gal's second
question on exposing her true feelings, I related back to the
union of marriage and how important it is to communicate
properly with our husbands. I certainly wouldn't expose
myself to *anyone* until I knew that it would be the man that I
marry. We do not want to be taken advantage of in any way,
be careful with what you share on dating relationships, often
times these relationships don't amount to anything. Use
discernment in all relationships, a woman usually has a pretty
good idea if she is with the man she will marry.

If we don't want to accept what our husbands are trying to
tell us, we hear only what we want to hear and miss out on
much of what he really said. We do this in the hopes that we
can scamper away from reality so we won't feel the hurt or
pain from what we just heard. Or we actually hear what was
said, but forget we ever heard it. This happens
subconsciously because we don't want to acknowledge what

the other person is saying and this is where severe communication breakdown in marriage can arise.

Intolerance of our husband's views and ideas stems from self-righteous thinking and is wrong. We're all entitled to our own ideas and opinions even between husband and wife. Too many times, we *think* we're right and our husband is wrong. But we all need the freedom to be oneself - think for oneself and to form opinions without criticism. The best thing we can do if we do disagree with our husband is first try and understand his feelings by validating his opinion if we can, and then state how we feel afterwards.

So what can you do next time you're in an argumentative debate with your husband? Well first, instead of butting in, like you always do, try taking the time to listen to what he has to say. As he talks put your brain muscle to work, and try walking in his shoes. When it is your turn to talk, you can tell him to put your shoes on his feet. It works ladies! Love the man you married. ♥

Reconnecting With Your Husband
17

What do you get when you pair two bulls together in one corral? An awful lot of head butting! A Marriage in this predicament will most likely head straight into the mud. All this means is couples need to pick themselves up out of the mud, stop butting heads with each other and start putting forth more effort in the reconnection department. Isn't your relationship worth it?

Remember your spoken thoughts at the altar as you looked into your husband's eyes, and swore to commit to him through thick and thin? If you feel disconnected from your man and feel like your not in a relationship anymore it is time to bring out that pre-marriage energy and get reconnected and re-bond totally with your husband.

Unfortunately, the culture of today makes the domestic diva *feel* deprived and worthless. Consequently more and more of these seemingly deprived women are jumping on the band wagon and establishing careers, leaving the husband and children to tend for themselves, leaving household duties and responsibilities unattended. How can couples in marriage be united when there are needs and desires that aren't getting met? How can couples profess to love each other when they are so busy doing the selfish things each wants? Outside opportunities and trivial desires keep couples from growing together in the marriage.

For example, a wife might have her own career, friends and agenda, which keeps her husband from wanting to get close to her, consequently he has his own buddies and sports games that he attends to, leaving his wife with her own agenda.

The husband in this scenario thinks his wife doesn't need, love or want him anymore, and when issues are challenged they both behave like two bulls, butting heads every chance they get. Neither spouse is involved with the other except for getting on each other's back because the lack of organization around the home. What chaos! Lack of household organization is great cause for neediness and disruption around the house.

It is a natural instinct for a "real man" to want to be in charge of the home and family, and to protect, love and care for his wife. But now-a-days many women feel they do not need this from a man, and rebel against it. This is very sad indeed for it is pushing away the design that God intentionally planned for marriage.

What happens when God's design gets messed with? It doesn't work out, plain and simple. Two bulls in one corral will cause tremendous head butting! No marriage can withstand the pressures of two bullies harassing each other. Nor can love be sustained when bulls go their separate ways either.

What can two bulls in marriage do? First off, remember the commitment you made with each other. Does that not mean something to you? Isn't it important to remain committed to what you started? Many important issues outside of marriage need a commitment as well to be successful. Commitments are like striving to reach our goals. If we don't put forth effort to attain the goals we make in life, they will probably not get accomplished. We have to work towards our goals to have them come to light.

Marriage is the same way; we women need to continue to put
forth effort to retain the love we once had in the marriage.
We have to work towards keeping the marriage built upon
the promise we made with our husband in the beginning for
the marriage to continue to shine bright in the darkness.

We do not have to be a bull to get our way, to feel
satisfied, or to be happy, we only have to stop being the bull
that we have been and start applying more effort into the
marriage.

Marriage is a never-ending journey. When wife shuts
down and stops' communicating is when she really loses
touch with her husband. The other communication problem I
see a lot is a wife not expressing her feelings to her husband
properly. Most of the time feelings get in the way and when
an angry bullying wife tries to communicate with her bullying
husband they head butt, by accusing, blaming and finger
pointing instead of talking. Those horns can play real nasty.

This is emotional abuse in the third degree. If we become
angry and hostile it will close our husband down and issues
will never get resolved. Here we go again, back to square one.
When issues don't get resolved they get stored away in the
mental capacities until a later date when they can be used to
justify the next heated argument. Move over, here comes, war
of the bulls!

Unresolved issues turn into resentment, which escalate
into more head butting. Pretty soon, because of this, and not
knowing how to communicate properly, wives eventually
learn to avoid issues they think will cause them to have
emotional outbursts with their husbands. They have finally
decided head butting doesn't work and so they shut down
totally. They feel it is better to just keep things the way they
are instead of confronting each other, which invariably causes
more frustration, resentment, animosity and pain.

The bottom line is if you want to feel married again and
be loved, learn to express feelings of anger appropriately
without accusing and blaming your husband for everything,
even if you know it is his fault. Try walking in your husband's

shoes for a change. Try putting forth a little bit more effort in the marriage like taking walks together, playing games, sharing a candle lit dinner, and whatever it is that you both enjoy. Try including your husband next time. Do it together! And of course, allowing God's wisdom and love into the marriage works wonders. Don't let your marriage turn into the loveless doldrums. Stop being so bullheaded and give in to each other for the sake of love and commitment! God will be pleased that you did. And remember, God's intention for marriage is a bull and a cow together in the corral, not two bulls. Love the man you married. ♥

Resentment - How It Can
Destroy Marriage
18

Resentment? What's that? According to Readers Digest Family Thesaurus, resentment means bad feelings, anger, outraged spirit, crossness, bad temper, dungeon huff, ill will, rancor, bitterness, sourness, wounded pride, hurt feelings, displeasure, animosity.

Do any of these feelings sound familiar? Do you harbor any of these feelings about your husband? This was one of my biggest faults when I was married. Before I discovered God's design for marriage, I piled up so much resentment within my psyche that my husband and I never got along. It's true, we do feel negative at times, and it is because we're hurting. We hurt because we allowed our husband to hurt us. We haven't learned to detach and so the hurt, hurts!

There is absolutely nothing wrong with you for having these kinds of feelings. What's wrong though, is when we harbor negative feelings inside of ourselves and don't do any thing about it. When we don't voice our feelings to our husband in a proper manner, or not at all, it will carry a negative affect on our self and those around us.

Love The Man You Married

Below are some prime examples of how not expressing our self properly will harbor resentment.

(1) A husband resents his wife for gaining weight. He pokes fun of her in front of their friends and sometimes won't make love to her. Because of his behavior, she thinks he doesn't love her anymore and she is hurt and resentful.

Jabbing fun at your wife because she has gained weight is cruel and demeaning. He needs to understand that she may lose weight for him, but eventually gain it all back because she didn't do it for herself. This husband needs to be told by the wife why she is gaining the weight back or why she is not losing the weight. And the husband needs to back off from his wife for a bit and let her decide for herself what needs to be done.

Ladies, our husbands are a bit naïve when it comes to knowing how to get what they want from us. That means we need to help them out a bit by telling them what we want, it's really that simple.

Here is what one of my newsletter readers told me about her husband spending time away from home and how she resented him.

I've been married for 14 years (with spouse for over 20 years in total). Everything we do revolves around him and I feel I've been neglected for 12+ years as he spends way more time with his friends than with me. So I told him this and now he wants to be with me all the time, but I resent that I had to tell him to spend more time with me and now I could care less if we do anything together. Now what do I do?

I told this gal she should enjoy this new time that she has found with the man she married. Do fun things together that you haven't done before, I said to her. Learn to like being with your husband more than your friends by making your husband your best friend. Let your husband see that he can enjoy his new time with you too.

Love The Man You Married

Sometimes we forget the fact that we're married because we have allowed ourselves to grow apart and away from the man we married. But it truly doesn't have to be like that. Didn't we marry the man we married because we loved him? We shouldn't look for ways to become unmarried. Another man isn't going to make us not feel a certain way. We make ourselves feel resentment and all the other negative ways we feel too. Let's learn to do something about it, we are in control of our happiness in the marriage and we can make it work!

(2) A wife is angry and resentful because her husband spends too much time with his buddies. When he finally does come home at night, she constantly nags at him about anything and everything and he ignores her and walks away feeling resentful.

Constantly complaining and nagging at your husband isn't going to bring him home any sooner. If you're going to nag, then it is often better to not say anything at all. If you're going to express your self nicely and assertively then by all means let the horn blow! But nagging is not going to work.

If your husband spends too much time out with his buddies that means it's time to get your mind occupied with something other than the fact your husband is out with his buddies instead of home with you. When he does come home, let him see you doing something you enjoy for yourself and that you aren't going to let his behavior bother you anymore. In other words, ladies, don't let your husband think you have nothing else better to do with your time, then sit around and brood over him. Continue on with the evening and forget about it. Afterwards, you'll feel so good about yourself you won't even feel resentful anymore!

Many issues like those above effect couples all the time. The goal here is to express how we feel about certain issues before they turn into resentment. Sometimes what happens is we choose to hold onto the hurt rather than express ourselves? Subconsciously we do this thinking we're actually getting our husband's back for something he did or didn't do. But in reality we're only causing more of an emotional problem within our self. And we don't want that.

A healthy, growing marriage relies on both couples feeling good about who they are. In that respect there is no room for that bad feeling called resentment.

Sometimes we blame our husbands for our feelings of resentment, and spend a lot of energy trying to change them into something we think will make us feel better about ourselves. But unfortunately, we find ourselves unfulfilled and wallowing in even more resentment because of it. This is so detrimental to the marriage. These feelings can literally cause us to think the grass is greener on the other side of the fence, but it is only a mirage, ladies, remember? The grass is not greener over there. In fact, our grass is green too, we just don't know it. Other women look at our grass and wish they had it. Don't let them get any closer. We take so much for granted and don't realize how blessed we really are. We are in control of our own marriage, and it's all up to us to cultivate it for our happiness. We have choices, and we're in charge of the outcome of our marriage!

The bottom line is we cannot change our spouse, and we cannot expect our spouse to make us happy! Know it and believe it!

Below I have compiled a small list of issues that can and will turn into resentment in the home. These things are only the branches that have their roots from the tree of life. The branches are dying parts of the tree that if not attended to like a baby needs milk will eventual shrivel up and die. Take care of your marriage.

The wife feels resentful because her husband...
spends too much money
spends too much time at work
spends too much time watching TV
flirtatious with other women

is controlling
is jealous
emotionally and mentally abusive
unhelpful around the house and with the kids

The husband feels resentful because his wife...
spends too much time at work
spends too much time with the kids
too religious
dresses better for others
spends too much money
gains weight
rejects him in bed
is controlling
flirtatious with other men

What you can do for yourself? These issues can be dealt with by proper communication and the willingness to forgive, detach and accept. Of course we cannot accept sinful behavior and if iniquitous behavior is going on in your marriage on a continual basis, then this does not apply. We need to clean up our act folks. Marriage cannot last when couples are carrying on in immoral behavior.

(1) Be assertive and express your feelings with a smile

(2) Forgive your spouse and let go of resentment you have towards them

(3) Communicate by listening more - ask questions

(4) Express true feelings without being afraid that you won't be loved

(5) Stop focusing on how to change your mate, but focus on how you can change yourself

(6) Find and nurture the spiritual aspect of your character

Number six entails greater understanding into the nature and design of God. In my book, *Journey on the Roads Less Traveled*, I explain the concepts associated with understanding the spiritual self and utilizing the spiritual tools that God has given us to nurture our self and spouse. For more information about this informative book, please see website: www.spiritual.journeybooks.4t.com ♥

Sermon on the Mount For Marriage
19

What do you think would happen between husband and wife if they committed themselves dutifully to following the characteristics of the Sermon on the Mount?

I think there would be way less divorce, how about you? Also, there would definitely be happier children in the household, wouldn't there?

Below I have made a one-week affirmation guide for marriage using the "Sermon on the Mount. Try it for one week, and if all goes well, try it for another week.

Copy/paste/print this weekly marriage guide out -- follow it for three weeks and see how you feel about yourself/husband.

1.) Today on Monday, I will not act proud with my husband. I will humble myself, even if I think I'm right.

How can we humble our self to our husband? Give in to them and let them be right? Why do we always have to be right? Why do we always have to get the last word in?

Blessed are the poor in spirit for their is the kingdom of heaven. Matthew 5:3

2.) Today on Tuesday, I will only please my husband, not myself. The whole day I will be sincerely gentle and kind to my husband. I will do only those things that would be giving and thoughtful to him.

Blessed are the meek for they shall inherit the earth. Matthew 5:5

3.) Today on Wednesday, I will give in to my husband's wishes. Whatever he asks, within reason will not be denied. I will not be self-seeking

4.) Today on Thursday, I will find one or more biblical ways to enhance my marriage. What would God want me to do for my marriage today? How can I make my husband feel good about who he is? How can I make him happy?

Blessed are those who hunger and thirst for righteousness, for they will be filled. Matthew 5:6

5.) Today on Friday, I will forgive my husband for wounding my heart. I will ask God to rid my heart and mind of negative feelings and resentment that I am feeling towards him. I will truly forgive.

Blessed are the merciful, for they will be shown mercy.
Matthew 5:7

6.) Today on Saturday, I will admit my faults to my husband and most importantly to God. Today I will ask God to grant me forgiveness and free me from the temptation to sin.

Blessed are the pure in heart, for they will see God.
Matthew 5:8

7.) Today on Sunday, I will be a peacemaker. I will not quarrel or fight with my husband. Today I will find one or more ways in which I can bring contentment and peace into my marriage.

Blessed are the peacemakers, for they will be called sons of God. Matthew 5:9

Do you think following the Sermon on the Mount for your marriage will be difficult to do? I don't think it will be. I think we can love the man we married every day! ❤

7 Reasons Why You Shouldn't Divorce The Man You Married

20

In this chapter I have identified seven triggers in marriage that are often used for justification for divorce, but really, none of these seven things warrant divorce or provide any validation what so ever to divorce the man you married.

1. You have a sexless marriage.

We don't want sex because we have lost touch with our husband! Essentially the bond that was there between us has been broken. When we spend too much time towards outside interests and wanting to be with friends we don't feel like getting sexy or even having sex with him!

Marriage needs attention! But we're giving that attention to our friends. It's true, woman usually give marriage the most attention, but we women are also more conscious of what needs our attention and consideration in the home. Face it ladies, we are more aware then men, and that is why God's specifically designed women to be in the home taking care of the logistics of the home instead of the man.

This is precisely why you should NOT break it off. You obviously need to spend more time together and get reacquainted like when you first married. You can't do that if you are ignoring your husband.

If your marriage is sexless or you are having sex infrequently it is time to bring romance back into the bedroom. You know what to do.

2. You constantly criticize your husband

If we often criticize and nag it is because we are expecting too much from our husband, and when things don't get done at the designated time, or in the exact way we would do it, we criticize and complain.

Faults become more apparent when expectations don't get met. We criticize our husband because we blame him for the disarray of the marriage. We notice all his faults, feel all his faults, and live all his faults. Essentially we are living in our husband's faults. No wonder we constantly criticize, we are too connected to the faults of our husband and so disconnected from the relationship of marriage! Learn to step out of the faults and into the marriage.

Hectic schedules can often make us come across as naggy and critical. It's because we're so stressed out! We want things done and think if we nag about it, it will get done. We're so busy that we don't have time to deal with the children, chores, cooking, career, and household. It is perfectly ok to delegate chores around the house to help lighten the load a bit. But what really needs to be done is to back off with the criticism and let our husband be who he is. This is all the more reason why we shouldn't break it off. Now is the perfect time to learn to accept our spouse for the way they are and stop trying to change things that we can't!

God certainly does not like that we criticize and disrespect who we married, and so the first action here would be to look at our self and see what it is that WE can do to change the situation to bring less negative attention towards our husband. Does it make you wonder why men like to be with their buddies all the time? Their buddies probably don't belittle them.

One gentleman reader was very concerned about his wife and her supposedly new found feelings for him. As I read his letter, my heart was breaking. Here is what he had to say.

My wife and me have been married for 20 yrs. About 3 weeks ago she stopped showing me affection. I'm not talking about sex. I confronted her about it and she said everything is bothering her. Her dad has Lou Gehrigs disease and her mother makes her feel guilty when we go away for a weekend. She also said she doesn't know if she has the right kind of love for me anymore. She also said she has been harboring pain for 20 years. That's funny she didn't show it. She goes to church every Sunday and I have started going back lately. I have never cheated on her and I told her I would not cheat. Any ideas?

Now doesn't that take the cake? I feel sorry for this poor man! How dispassionate was this woman. I felt as though the communication gap in this marriage was close to faltering. The wife in this dilemma reminded me of myself about ten years ago. The selfishness this woman displayed to her husband annoyed me to say the least. This marriage can be saved but they don't know it yet. I did tell this husband my ideas; here is what I told him.

Your wife is harboring resentment from past issues and they are obviously mounting up within her. Your wife needs an outlet for ridding her emotional issues. She really needs to forgive those who have hurt her. After she can forgive she can learn to set limits for herself so as not to allow others to hurt her again. Forgive, detach, be assertive, and love.

Your wife has a people pleaser personality. People pleasers tend to mask their true feelings and instead harbor unpleasant feelings later. Harboring negative feelings turn into resentment and bitterness. This is where your wife is right now. Her resentment has gotten out of hand so much that it is controlling her.

The good news is, your wife can be happy again and so

can you. But she has to be willing to make an effort on her part. Do you have any other spiritual outlets, such as bible study, and singing and praising to the Lord that you can do at home? Obviously she is not growing spiritually from going to Church. That means she is not getting what she needs. I believe that deep down your wife wants to grow out from her negative feelings but going to Church is keeping her from doing that. She is expecting a miracle from going to Church, but the miracle she needs comes from within herself.

As her husband, you should initiate Bible study in the home on a consistent basis. It will really help both of you connecting spiritually with God. It is when we become connected with Christ that we can humble ourselves and ask for forgiveness, and ask for His wisdom and love to guide our lives. Church is in our hearts and minds, and so "going" to church is not going to make a difference.

Your wife is calling out, but she is not calling out to God for help. Help her to call out to God. Be the man of the home.

3.) You often compare your husband to other men and you THINK your husband never measures up.

Comparing is wrong. When you compare in a negative way you are essentially telling your husband that they aren't good enough for you. It can lead to a poor self-image and make him feel weak as a man. Now how good can that be for his manly-hood? In the long run it leads to peer pressure type thinking because your husband feels he needs to continually challenge the person he is being compared to so he can prove that he is better in some way.

This is one way in which our negative feelings take control over our marriage and how we really perceive our husbands to be. If we see our husbands in a negative light it can make us want to compare them to other men. Everyone is different and as long as we continue to compare and expect our husband to change it will never happen. Our expectations once again will not be met and disappointment sets in. We really should never compare our man with other men in any way. Beauty is in the eye of the beholder. People are beautiful in their own way, faults and all. Be more accepting of those faults.

4.) You try to change your husband and it doesn't work

As a self help technique, try this for a change. Have your husband write down your bad habits, and the things that irritate him about you. Read them, study them, and change yourself! My husband did this to me once. Reality check!

5. You don't laugh anymore and it is impossible to have a lighthearted conversation.

Couples don't laugh anymore because of all of the above. Marriage needs attention. Marriage needs fun and games brought into now and again. What are you waiting for?

6. You THINK you are doing all the giving.

Are you keeping score? Pretend you're Santa Clause. Now check your "give list" for the week and see if your husband has been naughty or nice. If your husband has been nice to you this week, you will give him something special in the bedroom in return, but if he was naughty he can just forget about getting any sex at all from you, right?

Children all over the world are growing up understanding all about how to give conditional love like this and when they get married they can treat their own spouse conditionally like Santa did to them.

"No Dear, I'm not going to have sex with you tonight, you were mean to me all day today. Maybe tomorrow, if you're nicer to me."

Comedy shows like to depict this kind of behavior as being funny. This conditional sex-love dilemma in marriage is all about learning to give of your self unselfishly. Couples love each other selfishly because they do not have the knowledge to love properly. They love the way they have been taught to love. It is a conditioned and learned experience.

What does love mean to you? It doesn't have anything to do with the selfish arena. Love is not lust either, which frequently gets confused with love in the beginning stages of a romance and marriage. Love can sometimes take years to develop. Love is a process of learning through our spiritual and mental growth, and then giving of our self to our husband even when we don't FEEL like it. It is remembering to take action in those areas in our life that are, or should be important to us. Love is a development of ones self through the growing process, and then learning to practice that love with those we love.

In essence giving of one self is love, and we love others through giving. Giving comes from a heart and mind that is free of selfish precedents and self based love. This involves not just surrendering our sinful and selfish ways over to God, but allowing the Spiritual Christ into our heart and mind for emotional, and spiritual support. Without God's support in our marriage we would essentially utilize our self-seeking personality in the marriage, which in the long run cannot sustain a healthy and productive marriage.

7. You no longer feel good about yourself.

You don't feel good about your self, because you do not know your self. Low self-worth, depression and loneliness usually mean that we are not doing something in our life that we know we should be doing. We are not using all of our abilities to come to our potential. If we are living in a particular sin in our life and feel like we can't get out, that will keep us from coming to our full potential in marriage. Unfortunately when this happens in marriage, we tend to be overly needy with our husband by believing that they should make us FEEL happy and good about our self. But is this the responsibility of our husband?

It is through Jesus Christ that we learn to free ourselves from the weakness of sin. If we are living in sin, then we are not loving our self. If we don't feel good about ourselves, we certainly cannot love others; bitter and resent-filled hearts cannot love, it is impossible.

If we are living in our negative feelings, which many women do, we will not know the fulfillment of knowing what "real love" is. I thrived on my negative feelings. I felt it was the only way I could ever get a point across to my husband but now when I look back on those days, I see how unhealthy my attitude was because of my destructive feelings.

Now ladies, did you know that by surrendering your guilt, resentment, angry feelings, and sin to God it would free you from behaving selfishly and rebelliously toward your husband? Essentially it is when you let go of the bitterness in your heart that you learn to love properly. This is called surrendering to love because God is love!

Here is how it works, we give up the weakness that has been taking over our life, and we finally grow spiritually into a new person in Christ. That is when we learn to love who we are, and also loving others freely without negative feelings tearing at our flesh.

This issue of low self worth is the root to all of the above issues. This is why I stress constantly in all of my articles, newsletters, and books, "that we need to take care of our selves first"!

Taking care of our self is the toughest challenge most of us face on a daily basis, whether it is in our marriage or other relationship with people. If we ourselves are in need of love and life, we certainly cannot give love or life to another.

Remember that none of these issues warrant breaking it off, they do warrant however, putting forth more effort in those areas that need our attention. And that is precisely why you shouldn't break it off. Surrender and love the man you married! ♥

Romancing Your Marriage
21

Bring out the creative person you are and splash some good old fashion fun back into your marriage! You can do these things right from home without breaking the pocketbook. Turn the TV off, play some of your favorite music and do some enjoyable things together for a change. Watch the relationship between you and your husband get tighter!

1. Play a board game instead of watching TV (scrabble, monopoly, Clue)
2. Listen to some Jazz music, light some candles and talk about anything
3. Have a romantic picnic
4. Get on the floor together and do stretch exercises
5. Take turns reading a book that you both like out loud, and then discuss what you read.
6. Make your own home movie or music CD
7. Create a personal web page together

8. Cook a scrumptious meal together
9. Buy a microphone and have your own karaoke
10. Give each other a twenty minute massage, and see what happens

Here are a few things you can do, if you have time, and money in the wallet.

1. See a live play at the theater
2. Go to the beach or mountains for the weekend or longer if permissible
3. Take up a hobby together, such as sailing or photography
4. Spend the night in a hotel. (Make sure they have a Jacuzzi)
5. Take up roller skating or ice skating (fun way to keep those legs in shape)

Sensuality and passion between you and the man you married can become heightened when you share in fun and enjoyable things together. We're always learning, growing and noticing new things about the man we married, even after twenty years of marriage! They change, we change, and they grow, and as we share stimulating and interesting times with our spouse so does our perception of them change in a way we didn't think possible. And this is why we shouldn't let our marriage become dreary and mundane but always seek out fun and challenging things to share together in the growth process of marriage.

It's true; we do change as we experience life and as we get older but were not different people. Hopefully we'll get smarter, more experienced, happier, and more fun loving as we age.

Did you know that couples that grow spiritually and mentally together instead of apart have better marriages? It's true!

Don't feel intimidated to try something different from your usual routine. You can literally get so caught up in your daily routine that you miss out on the special opportunities to add a little pack of spunk into your marriage.

This is also true in the lovemaking department. Try different techniques and different positions. There is no need to be shy with your husband, more than likely he too, would like to try something different in the bedroom.

Come on; don't let your marriage dry out! If you feel like your marriage is heading into the doldrums and you can't get out of the rut, then its time to share more of your self with your husband. Why wait for you to both get bored with the relationship? Play together! Surprise your husband with a live musical dance wearing something very skimpy.

Did you know that just doing simple things together could bring laughter and joy back into your conversations? Sharing pleasurable times together will not only bring you closer with your husband but will help you to remember who your husband is by helping to reconnect the bonds that have been severed between you.

Often times, because of busy schedules and different agendas, couples don't realize how easy it is to grow apart, until one day down the road they don't know each other anymore. Over the course of time, months or years, a growth process takes place, and you find that the man you married has changed because you have not grown together, but apart, and that's not good!

So turn off that TV, and get to know each other again through sharing of yourself. Above all, while doing these things together, remember to always share the best part of yourself with your husband--your love!

There is no better gift of love that you can give your husband then your willingness to accept him just the way he is. Men need this acceptance from their wives and they need reassurance from time to time that you still love them, especially if the two of you have grown apart. Acceptance is love, and by showing open-mindedness, understanding and patience with your husband, your marriage can endure through the hard-hitting times as well as the enjoyable. ♥

Love the Person You Are and Hate the Person You've Been

22

I devote this chapter to focusing on and changing our self. Maybe it is our attitude that we need to change or maybe it is our feelings. Whatever it is that needs changing let's start examining the real person we are so we can begin to hate the person we have been.

Did you know that love is a choice? We choose to love or not to love. It's that simple. But I believe the non-loving choice is not our "true selves." The non-loving self is absorbed in anger, judgment, resentment, and all kinds of things that we allow to control how we love. This is because we haven't let go of past hurts. These hurts control who we are and how we react to people around us. The bottle controls an alcoholic and a hurting person is controlled by resentment.

My husband used to tell me, "I love you, but I don't love the disease." What he meant was that he loved me for who I really was, not the alcoholic. The alcoholic in me couldn't love either. I was selfish and cold. I couldn't give of myself to my husband because I was too needy living inside of my addiction. My thinking was distorted to the point that I actually thought that it was him who needed to give more of himself to me! Boy was I way out in left field, and blind to boot.

In essence, this is how we allow feelings and thoughts to

control how we will love, and when we will love. The person who is controlled by their feelings is unable to fully love another person. Unfortunately so, many of us are restricted from ever loving properly because of negative feelings. This is why I stress how important it is to watch out for what we allow into our hearts and minds!

Even in our own marriage some of us are incapable of giving any love until we decide to give up our position that our way is the right way, and the only way! Feelings make us see things in our husband that causes us to scrutinize the person he is. But ladies, trying to dissect our husband's feelings and experience them as our own doesn't help the love process.

Most couples when they profess to love each other, it is what they imagine them to be, not what they are. This is phony love and phony self. It's not real. Knowing this we can see how important it is to love ourselves first. That way we can actually love another and be real. Loving our husband means to give something of our self to him, right? To give is to love and to love is to give. It's really so simple. And I think we should be giving more of who we really are to our husband even when we don't feel like it! And so how do you like them apples?

On the flip side of the coin, we shouldn't change to be what our husband wants us to be either. If we do that, we'll become a clone of who they are, how boring! We would also resent the fact that we are only trying to please our husband and not our self. If we change to be just what our husband wants then we have become a people pleaser. Well, let me tell you this. People pleasers are the biggest resentment protectors in the world. I know this because I was a resentment propagator for a long time in my marriage until I learned to grow out from destructive feelings and myself.

Ladies, we should change to be what we really are! Our ability for love and to love is much greater then we allow. We are afraid to be ourselves so much that we strive to be what our husband wants from us, even when deep down that is not what we want or need.

So what keeps the real you from coming out in the open with your real feelings is the emotional baggage called resentment. Bitterness and anger will linger in the heart for years, if you allow it to, because you are unable to forgive and then forget.

When we don't forgive what happens? When we cannot forgive properly it causes shame, guilt and anger within us, and then we become emotionally overstressed with our husband, which limits our own "love capacity" to be what God intended for it to be.

It is so true that what we "generate into our heart will come out in our actions." Our capacity to love is how true we are to ourselves. We certainly aren't very true to ourselves or to God when we are unable to forgive our husband. When we do forgive our husband completely and unconditionally, as God forgives us, then we no longer experience the past hurts. We feel freer to be ourselves and to be more in control of who we are. With that, the spiritual growth process begins to kick in and we indeed experience love, even to those who are cruel to us or don't love us at all. You see it doesn't really matter what others think of us, what does matter is what we think of our self.

Being able to truly forgive completely is a courageous act in itself. Forgiving enables us to see that we do have the strength with God's help to deal with our emotions and feelings on our own. When we decide to forgive from the goodness of our heart, we will learn to be who it is God intended us to be, and to love who we are. We won't need to carry the burden of another's failings in our heart.
So ladies, you can choose to love. Don't be afraid to forgive your husband. Forgive and love your husband and all others whom you are associated with. Real love comes through acceptance and forgiveness. And when you have forgiven completely all of the people you need to forgive, you can finally be free to love the person you are, and hate the person you've been. ♥

116

Don't Allow Negative Emotions To Control Your Marriage
23

Emotions play a big role in our life. They are active and alive twenty-four hours a day, even in our dreams. Emotions literally tell us what to do with our marriage, family, job, career, self, and how we love others. If we don't control the course that our emotions run, we might be heading down the road towards destruction.

Are you allowing your negative emotions to control your marriage? When was the last time you got angry? What do you do when your friend turns her back on you? What do you do when your husband disrespects you? What do you do when your children continue to misbehave? What happens if your emotions tell you that you don't love your husband anymore? What are you going to do? Do you let jealousy and resentment tell you what to do in certain circumstances?

Before we can understand the full potential of our self and our emotions we need to understand a little bit about who we are, and why we do and say the things we do. How do we handle our selves with certain issues and particular circumstances? What do we do when conflict rears its ugly head in our marriage? We get emotional, right? We lash out

117

with anger, or we clam up in resentment, or express our self improperly. Are we letting our emotions rule our marriage, our self, and our life?

Most of us, in some way or another, let our destructive emotions control us. We have a hard time giving things over to God, even though it is what He instructs us to do. Why do you think that is? Why does God not let us live the way we want? I think it is because we are imperfect here on earth? Our own understanding is off course. Meaning, we do imperfect things? We error, we sin, we become angry, we disrespect the ones we love the most, we lie, some of us cheat, steal, and then some of us do really bad things, all because we are imperfect people.

God wants us to give to Him our imperfections and He will make things right in His way. God doesn't want us to use our feelings to do unconstructive things, but constructive things. As you all have come to know, we have good emotions and bad emotions. Some of us women are more emotional than others, and we use those feelings to control who we are. But this stunts the growth process, and causes all kinds of problems for our loved ones. First of all, understand it's okay to have feelings, and to even get angry, but how we express, or don't express that anger is the key here. It can make or break a marriage or relationship in the long run.

The problem is that some days we just feel like crap (pardon the slang). We feel so much like crap that everyone around us gets treated like crap! You know the feeling. What's happening is we are letting our emotions control the person God intended us to be. We have so much potential in us just waiting to come out, and yet, we haven't submitted our bitter and resent filled person over to God, instead we have decided, selfishly, I might add, to handle situations under our own understanding of things. But what do we know?

Here is what one reader shared with me after reading one of my articles about controlling our emotions.

Love The Man You Married

After having a terrible argument with my wonderful husband this morning, and hearing things from his mouth that left me feeling deserted, I turned to your article called "Understanding Our Emotions". Your article hit the nail on the head in several ways. I haven't even finished reading the article but I needed to tell you the peace that began to wash over me. Congratulations on opening your heart to God and fulfilling a purpose He has for you through writing. I'm anxious to read more of your articles. Thanks again! Be blessed and receive.

I believe the peace this woman was feeling was in her ability to understand how important it is that we do give God those feelings that are imperfect. Even though we are imperfect people doesn't mean we have a right to treat others with our destructive emotions? This woman's peace was found through her own realization of knowing she can let it all go by giving it to God. It is in hearing these words from others that I become more aware of God working in people's lives through the power of the Holy Spirit.

By freeing our self of unwanted emotions and negativity that normally upset and confuse our husband we become the giving and loving wife we were meant to be. In essence those of us who haven't learned to be attuned with the spiritual aspect of our character are still letting our negative emotions impact the way we behave towards our husband and others in our life. This is why we get angry and disrespectful, maybe even violent towards those we love. We literally filled up with negative emotions.

Why do you think people are selfish? Selfishness stems from neediness. We are needy because our emotions are not fixing the problems in our life and marriage. Anger, bitterness, resentment, disrespect, pride selfishness, rebelliousness, these things do not fix our marriage, family, or how we feel inside. They just keep piling up! The more our crappy emotions pile up the more selfish we become. It is a never-ending story!

How can bitterness and resentment control us, you may ask? Resentment is just another way of thinking. Resent-filled thinking is very flawed to say the least. I know these things; I lived in my resentment for almost a decade, even though I didn't know it at the time. Resentment told me not to forgive my husband. It told me to look for my husband's faults and dissect his personality. This error in thinking kept me from growing out from self and being happy in my marriage. I literally lived in my emotions.

Believe me when I say, emotions can wreck havoc in your life. Emotions might tell us it is okay to have affairs, to steal, cheat, lie, do drugs, or treat our husband with disrespect and contempt. But that is not who we really are?

All that needs to be done here is to discover the spiritual aspect of our character and grow more into the loving nature of our Creator. We do that by giving up the old emotional selfish person over to God and ask Him to fix us. The bible tells us that Jesus Christ left us His Spirit of Truth and Wisdom. If we listen to Truth and Wisdom it will fix us! It really will!

"We have not received the spirit of the world but the Spirit who is from God, that we may UNDERSTAND WHAT GOD HAS FREELY GIVEN US!" The man without the Spirit does not accept the things that come from the Spirit of God, for they are foolishness to him, and he cannot understand them, because they are spiritually discerned." 1 Corinthians 2:10-14

Do you understand what God has freely given you? This is the question that we need to understand and answer. Some of us already understand, and that is why we have already chosen to be a part of God's family, and because of that, we now have the potential within us to grow out from our emotions, and into a better way to love and accept others, which is from a spiritually based standpoint. We have increased spiritual awareness within our personality by freeing old pains and past hurts, giving them to God. And the awesome thing about it, we don't even have to get all

120

religious over it! Because when we realize the spiritual potential within us, we actually start applying God's spiritual tools into our marriage, career, job, family, children, and whatever else we do in life. This is not something religious, but something spiritual.

Those who believe in Christ's death and resurrection and put their faith in Him will know all they need to know to be free to love, free to be who they are, and free to just be! God has revealed it to them by His Spirit -- the Holy Spirit. ♥

The Sexually Satisfied Marriage

24

Marriage is like a tricycle. One of the back wheels is the mental (emotional) area in marriage, another back wheel is for the physical (sexual), and the front wheel, which is the leader, is for the spiritual aspects of the marriage. If one of these facets of marriage is missing, what is going to happen? The marriage is going to be unbalanced and topple over.

Did you know that your feelings could affect your sexual appetite? For instance, if you're feeling bitter, resentful, or guilty towards your spouse, you won't feel like having sex with them. Should we deprive our spouse of sex because of how we are feeling? I don't think so.

It is not right to deny our spouse the sexual fulfillment that marriage so much needs just because we're mad at them or we're having a bad day. Nothing could be further from the truth.

Feelings of bitterness are caused by an unforgiving attitude. An unforgiving attitude is what holds us back. It is what keeps us living in the past and not looking towards the future. Jesus said we are to forgive seventy times seven…forgiving properly means that we don't harbor the pain anymore, and that means we don't bring up the issue with our spouse again! Period!

Ladies, we are in control when it comes to the sexual aspects of the marriage. Learn to use that to your advantage. After having sex is the best time to discuss any issues that are bothering you. Be nice, and express yourself lovingly and appropriately. Don't nag and complain.

Many couples don't discuss their sexual preferences with each other. But this is not the time to be shy either. It's very vital to the sexual health of the marriage that couples express their pleasures in the bedroom arena. Both need to know and be acquainted with the zones and parts of the body, which are capable of producing pleasurable sensations.

Below are a few guidelines to take note of for a great sensual and passionate marriage, even after ten, and twenty years of marriage!

1. Allow spouse the freedom to be who they are. Be understanding and considerate of their feelings at all times, not just in the bedroom.
2. Communicate any sexual issues and problems that have developed in the marriage. Let go of your sexual inhibitions and express your pleasures in the lovemaking arena. Ladies, men like to give pleasure to their wives, so now is your chance to speak up and tell him what you like.
3. Thank God everyday that you are married to a person who is willing to discuss and express these issues with you.
4. Always be loving and available. Sometimes we women just aren't in the mood. But it doesn't matter; give yourself to your husband anyway, unless you are sick or going through menstruation.
5. Create an appealing bedroom that you both like. Redecorate it with tasteful decor that you both have picked out.

6. Make yourself attractive and pleasing to each other. Buy a new skimpy nightgown, and men buy some bikini briefs. If you already wear that kind of under clothing, buy some silky cartoon boxers - something different that you wouldn't normally wear.
7. Be romantic and loving. Light some aromatic candles for a sensual and romantic atmosphere.

This is for the ladies reading this. I have learned through my own marriage that our men NEED to have sex. Some men like it everyday, others every other day, while others maybe two times a week. Be ready when your husband wants to have sex. Don't reject your husband for just any reason; make him feel loved and good about himself. Men love this kind of sensual pampering.

When we reject our husband, that is when they begin THINKING about looking elsewhere to find fulfillment, and we don't want that, do we ladies? So often we take our husband for granted in this area, and don't realize the importance of sexual fulfillment for the man in our life. Don't give your man any reasons to look elsewhere, take care of the man you married!

"The wife's body does not belong to her alone, but also to her husband. In the same way, the husband's body does not belong to him alone but also to his wife. Do not deprive each other except by MUTUAL consent and for A TIME, so that you may devote yourselves to prayer. Then come together again so Satan will not TEMPT you because of your lack of self-control. 1 Corinthians 7:4-6

Okay men, your turn, the most important thing you can do for your wife is to not rush into the lovemaking act in 30 seconds. Come on now, be more considerate. You know it takes your wife a bit longer than you. Tell her how much you love her, and rub her all over, wherever she likes it. Be more patient in the bedroom, your time will come soon enough.

124

Bottom line is do not deprive or reject each other! A happy sexual relationship involves right attitudes. It is God's will that married couples enjoy sexual relations with each other. Find out what wheel is missing in your marriage and fix it. ♥

Gods Rock Solid Truths
For Your Marriage
25

A healthy marriage always relies on the foundation of honesty, trust, honor, respect and commitment. These rock solid truths are found in the bible. What are rock solid truths? God designed marriage to be indissoluble. The only disclaimer there is for marriage is if there is physical violence and any sort of continual abuse going on. The latter is debatable, but Gods rock solid truths are not. In other words, these are not my opinions or beliefs, but Gods.

Should adultery be included in the disclaimer for divorce? I don't think so. What is adultery? It is a spiritual imbalance of one or both spouses who are unable to commit themselves to one another. The root of major issues in marriage originates from an unhealthy spiritual psyche.

The truth is if a husband who cheats on his wife wants to be justified in his adulterous affairs he needs to go to a shrink. God's design for marriage does not justify adultery as a means for divorce. If a husband is willing to discontinue in his weakness and seek Jesus Christ for his marriage, then a wife should not look to divorce her husband over it. God wants both spouses to support the marriage pledge by His foundations of rock solid truths. We are to honor and respect our spouse for who they are, faults and all. A healthy marriage maintained by Gods truths will enable couples to respect and honor one another. Commitment is a word that means so much to God, but yet, so little to couples in their marriage. If couples were committed to their marriage they would be looking for reasons to stay together instead of reasons to leave each other!

I recently confronted my husband of 5 years about his adulterous affair. I needed guidance on forgiveness and how to get rid of the anger, rage and hurt that the affair has caused within me. Your E-books and articles on forgiveness were very informative and helpful with many scriptures to keep in my spiritual bank. I want to save my marriage, and I thank you for having the courage to write such an unconventional newsletter. We live in unconventional times and it helps to know that Christian material is available for all types of marital problems.

Unconventional newsletter? I wouldn't necessarily say that my newsletters are unconventional. I write from a biblical standpoint, not from a worldly view, therefore, I suppose anyone who doesn't read or know Gods word would call my newsletter and e-books unconventional. But Gods words NEVER change! God's rock solid truths are here to stay forever! She is right though; some people do live in unconventional times. It is those people who find it hard to maintain certain spirituality for them selves and marriage.

What we need to do is stop looking at the grass on the other side of the fence. If you keep looking at it, soon enough you will see the brown spots where the dog has urinated.

Love doesn't even factor into any of this. People use the word "love" a bit too loosely. "I love you." What does that mean? Show me you love me and I will believe you. Give to me without wanting anything in return. Die for me if you have to. Don't say, "I love you", show me that you love me!

The truth many women perceive to be correct for their

marriage comes from self. The self guided tour for marriage believes in divorce, infidelity, addiction, resentment, hate, lust, bitterness of heart and immorality, etc. If we believe these truths long enough, what happens? We become dead to the rock solid truths that come from God and remain in bondage to the sinful nature of self. We are looking out into the world for our marriage answers, but the world doesn't have the answers we need, in fact, the world supports divorce. What kind of thinking is that?

The worldly woman believes the only way out of an unhappy marriage is divorce. And isn't it ironic how society has made it so justifiable to divorce over such pettiness. The spiritually bankrupt psyche expects happiness and contentment at all costs, and will go after it with gusto through the only understanding they know; foundation of self. The feminist movement is run like this. More and more women are joining the ranks of this movement because they have each other for support and validation. But those women are wearing rose-colored glasses, ladies. Everything looks and sounds right and glamorous, but it isn't. The rosy colored glasses have blurred their sight, and dampened their hearing. Satan hands out these rose colored glasses to all who will accept them. I wore rose-colored glasses for several years in my own marriage. For about ten years I thought I had it all right. After a time, I thought to myself, "Now can this be all there is? If I have it all so right, why do I feel so rotten?"

Ironically, the sinful nature even acknowledges the existence of God, but doesn't have faith enough to pursue the rock solid truths for marital happiness and contentment. All of this error in thinking can be eliminated from the psyche. The way we think, what we believe, and what we allow into our heart and mind undeniably comes back out in the way we live, and how we direct our marriage. We live what we think. In retrospect, what we generate into our heart comes out in our actions. Acknowledging just isn't enough. We also need to accept it (God). We need to stop looking out into the world for the answers for our life; they just don't have the answers we need. God has the rock solid answers!

Because most women do not know any better, they end up playing god in their marriage, and in so doing, do those things which come from the selfish arena, which are in contradiction to Gods rock solid truths. For an example, if I play god, I will direct my marriage under my own understanding of what *I want and what I feel.* The selfish aspect of my nature tells me to do what I want, and to do what will make *me* happy, not considering the feelings of my husband.

Culture of society plays itself out with this kind of error in thinking. People are like chameleons, individuality is lost, and becomes one in its beliefs. The world acknowledges that God exists, but can't seem to accept the Godly truths for themselves. As a matter of fact, the world is trying hard to eliminate God from many of the issues and components of life that at one time were paramount.

In whom the God of this world hath blinded the minds of them which believe not, lest the light of the glorious gospel of Christ, who is the image of God, should shine unto them. 2 Corinthians 4:4

The bottom line is the word of God is open and revealed to everyone, except for those who refuse to believe. Satan "is the god of this age" His work is to deceive, and he has blinded those who don't believe in Jesus Christ.

For such are false apostles, deceitful workers, transforming themselves into the apostles of Christ. And no marvel; for satan himself is transformed into a angel of light. 2 Corinthians 11:13-14

Satan and his servants deceive married couples by appearing to be attractive, good, and moral. Many unsuspecting marriages follow these smooth talking, bible quoting leaders and are lead into the practice of immorality, lust and deceit. Such as the practice of divorce, homosexuality, infidelity, and other immoral acts has become a thing of this new culture in the world. You and your marriage do not have to be a part of it. Don't allow yourselves to be lead astray with all of the other marriages, save yours now by bringing your marriage under the foundations of God's design, and love the man you married!

The biggest and greatest truth is Gods rock solid truths never change. They always stay the same even when cultures around the world change to conform to immorality of the day, God's words and precepts stay the same.

God intends marriage to be a lifetime commitment. That being the case, those entering into marriage, should never consider divorce an option for solving problems or a way out of a relationship that only *seems* like it is dead. Your marriage can be restored. It really can! ❤

"…That he which made them at the beginning made them male and female, and said, "For this cause shall a man leave father and mother and shall cleave to his wife; and they twain shall be one flesh? Wherefore they are no more twain, but one flesh. What therefore what God hath joined together, let not man put asunder. Mathew 19: 3-6

How to Have The Right Attitude
For Your Marriage

26

Did you know that your attitude in life could make or break your marriage? It's true! Your attitude tells you what to do in certain situations and how to behave with specific issues in your marriage. Are you carrying around the right attitude for your marriage? This chapter explores several reasons why you might be carrying around the "not so right attitude" for your marriage.

1. Do you have a positive attitude about God? Attitudes reflect what you feel about God. Meaning your whole outlook on life can be transformed into a positive experience if you have a deep and meaningful relationship with your Creator. You do this by getting to know Him and by "wanting" to understand God's wisdom filled ways more than your ways.

You ought to really try to love God with all of your heart, mind and soul and God will give you the faith and confidence you need to be loving and compassionate to the man you married. This doesn't just apply to marriage. This application applies to all the people, friends, and family that you are associated with.

That's all about it! A simple exchange takes place between you and God. When you trust in Him, He'll then give you the wisdom you need for your life and marriage.

2. Do you let your husband dictate what your attitude will be? Many of us do that. Remember were like chameleons. We listen to the negative attitudes of our husband and it rubs off on us. He turns green and we turn green. This is what happens in marriage when couples become entangled in a heated argument.

These kinds of arguments usually don't get anywhere because they are being played off with bad attitudes. Your husband says something negative about you and you in turn look for something bad to say about him. What needs to be done is to start thinking positive about God in your life and marriage, and your negative attitude will vanish from your mind!

3. Is your attitude in marriage consistent with your actions? In other words, your mind and heart must know, see, and feel the same way, not in contradiction to each other or you will come off as a hypocrite.

If you try and be something that you are not, it will eventually come out in your actions. Your heart has to feel what you say, and you mind must know what it is your heart wants. Otherwise, you might speak things that are not true to your husband and come off as hypocritical with him.

This happens because you are getting the wrong messages sent to you by the culture of society. The culture of today believes it is ok to lie to your husband and to commit adultery, but what does your heart say? We need to put 100 percent attitude into our marriage by loving our marriage with all our heart, mind and soul. That's what commitment is all about!

The same thing is true with our attitude about God. He wants us to love him not just with our mind, but with our heart and soul too.

These people honor me with their lips, but their hearts are far from me. They worship me in vain; their teachings are but rules taught by men. Matthew 15:8-9

4. Is your attitude about your marriage causing you to sin? Are your thoughts and feelings getting in the way of your actions? Have you taken your eyes off the spiritual Christ for your marriage? Or maybe you "need" the spiritual Christ for your marriage.

To see your marriage in the positive light, and to understand why some things happen the way they do, or why you might feel a certain way all comes down to what you believe is right and good for your marriage.

By reading your articles and (e-books) I realize how much I lack wisdom going into any relationship. But I am grateful to God that God is preparing me as a better partner for the future relationship through your ministry. I see God already working out and testing out some of your principles in my life, and I see God moving my life directing and guidingthis special relationship in my life right now.

I would love to read more of your articles and books, so please continue to educate young people like myself and save us from further headaches.

Wisdom definitely takes the right attitude so we can understand it with the spiritual clarity it deserves. After all, some thoughts of wisdom *seem* like wisdom but really isn't wisdom at all. This is how people fall into worldly traps of society. Satan deceives! The wisdom you are reading in this book is not my wisdom, it comes from God, I'm just the messenger girl.

The right attitude isn't afraid to love God wholly. The right attitude is not afraid to be humble and meek in front of others. The right attitude is the spiritually happy attitude. That is the wisdom that has been given us, yet most of us don't use that wisdom in our own marriage.

If we do not trust God for the marital guidance that our marriage needs, who are we going to trust? Our self? Society? Culture? What do they know? Where does their judgment for "your marriage" come from? God wants you to love him enough that you will build your marriage upon His foundation of wisdom and truth.

Therefore, everyone who hears these words of mind and puts them into practice is like a wise man who built his house on the rock. The rain came down, the streams rose, and the winds blew and beat against the house; yet it did not fall, because it had its foundation on the rock. But everyone who hears these words of mine and does not put them into practice is alike a foolish man who built his house on sand. The rain came down, the streams rose, and the winds blew and beat against the house, and it fell with a great crash. Matthew 7:24-27

5. Do you know how to recognize God's positive results in your marriage?

A good tree always bares good fruit, which becomes noticeably apparent to everyone. When you finally give up "your way" for "God's way" your attitude begins to change, and you will start to feel better about your self. You become a tree of abundance for your marriage. Here is how it works. Your marriage that you may have thought was dead has been brought to life by your attitude. Your whole outlook and position in the marriage will transform into an optimistic and constructive way of thinking. This happens because you have trusted in God for the care of your marriage. Your marriage now stands on the foundation called the rock. When the rain and winds came, and blew dangerously against your house, your attitude saved it from falling. Way to go!

6. Do you know how to keep allowing God's life force in your marriage? Never lose sight of who you are. You are a child of God and God is your source, not society nor culture but The Omnipotent God! Open your eyes and start seeing with the wisdom that God has given you.

    a. Imitate Christ's forgiving attitude
    b. Let God's love guide your life
    c. Let the peace of Jesus rule in your heart
    d. Keep God's word in your heart at all times

This is the wisdom Gods children inherit when they have trusted in Him. Your positive attitude and outlook on life can now love God with all your heart, mind and soul. And because you have shown you love God by trusting in Him, he has given you the spiritually positive attitude for your marriage. ♥

Therefore as God's chosen people, holy and dearly loved, clothe yourselves with compassion, kindness, humility, gentleness, and patience. Bear with each other and forgive whatever grievances you may have against one another. Forgive as the Lord forgave you. And over all these virtues put on love, which binds them all together in perfect unity. Galatians 3:12-14

How To Treat Your Man Like A Man?
27

Are you a controlling wife? Do you take your husband for granted? Most women don't realize it but they abuse their husbands daily just by their actions. Many women of today feel that marriage revolves solely around them and their husband's are supposed to give them everything their heart desires.

If we aren't getting what we want from our man could it be because we are not treating our man like a man? Stop pushing him around and he'll come around.

1. Don't undermine your husband's decision making

This is a biggy in marriage. Isn't it true that we women want things our way! We have been taught from grade school to go after our dreams and aspirations in life no matter what the consequences, even if that means rejecting our husband's needs and wishes. We do what WE want and what WE need.

Love The Man You Married

Why would a woman of today be so determined to chip away at her husband's manly authority and advice?

Face it ladies, we haven't exactly helped to make our man feel like a man. If we don't accept the man we married, why would we expect to get what we want from him? If we are rejecting, blaming, controlling, demeaning, undermining, and complaining about our husbands we certainly aren't respecting the man we married. If we weaken our husband's manly resolve what's left but our feminist attitude and bossy selfish egos? Are we taking the man we married for granted? I think we are and that's what's killing marriage!

How do I know all this? I used to undermine my husband all the time. I wouldn't let him be the man of the house. I was bossy and rebellious. I want you to know what I have come to know. It's great! Let's take a look at some of the improper actions we take with the man we are supposed to love.

2. Don't reject your husband

How many times last month did you tell your husband that you were too tired or had a headache or simply shrugged him off because you were mad at him? Probably more times then you really think. Shouldn't we want to satisfy our husband's needs every single day, regardless, whether we feel like it or not? We women need to please and satisfy the men we're married to and we'll get our hearts desire. We really will!

3. Give your husband space (freedom)

Do you complain because your husband likes to have free time away with the guys? Maybe you feel he should be home doing chores or watching the children on his day off. But face it ladies, our man deserves time away to be with his friends to play golf, fish or hunt, or whatever it is he does just as much as we deserve to be with our friends.

Did you know that a husband that is allowed the freedom to be with his buddies is a happier and more content filled man? Isn't that what we want anyway? Yes it is. We want our husbands to be happy and content being with us, their wives. All we need to do is give them some freedom to be, and they come back respecting us more for trusting in them.

4. Cook your husband hot and nutritious meals every day

It is so true that one way to our man's heart is through his stomach. Ask any man and he'll tell you. I know that some of you ladies who work out of the home just don't have the time to cook nice meals everyday. The solution to that is simple. Buy your self a crock-pot and a crock-pot cookbook and learn to make delicious homemade meals with it. Crock-pot cooking is so simple and tasty to boot. You throw all the ingredients in the pot and it cooks safely all day, and the food will be ready when you both come home from work. The time is saves us in the kitchen is noteworthy. Every kitchen should have a crock-pot.

5. Respect your husband

What's so hard about respecting the man we married? You wouldn't believe how often we disrespect our husbands without even knowing it!

Here are some ways in which we control the marriage and disrespect our husbands. When we think he can't do anything as good as we can, we certainly won't be able to respect him, right? Is treating your husband like one of the children respecting him? Is complaining about his faults respecting him? Is telling him what he's going to do respecting him? Is rejecting him sexually respecting him? Is belittling him respecting him? Well then, stop doing all these things and you are on your way to respecting the man you married.

6. Let your husband protect you

God made man to be the protector of women. Men love to do it, they want to do it, and they feel like a man when we let them do it. But most married women don't feel they need protected because they can take care of themselves. They carry mace, a gun and take karate classes and act like a man and still, they are getting beaten, raped, manhandled, and murdered. If a woman is married why on earth would she want to take away her husbands god-given natural abilities as her protector?

A married woman needs to allow her husband to do his job in the manner in which he does it best, by protecting and loving his wife with the natural abilities God gave him. How can a man do that when the woman won't let him? This is how a man loves his woman!

Seriously now, it's really that simple. What happens when we don't allow our husbands to protect us? We reject their love for us. Don't you want to be loved by your man? Did you know that when we don't let our husband's love us the way God meant for a man to love his wife, we are rebelling against God?

Come on, ladies let your husband take care of you the way that comes natural to him.

7. Submit to your husband (love God)

Ladies, first you must learn to submit to God. This was a major issue in my marriage for many years because I didn't accept God. I was looking out into the world for the answers to my marriage problems when the answers were within my spiritual self the whole time. I finally grew to accept and love God. That is the root of submitting right there.

By growing out from the selfish person I was, I learned to understand what submitting to my husband was all about. Once a woman learns to submit to her husband she will see that by submitting she is actually in more control of her marriage and a better marriage wife because of it. In other words, a woman will not lose anything of her self by submitting but will gain more of herself that was lost. ♥

"Now I want you to know that the head of every man is Christ, and the head of the woman is man, and the head of Christ is God." 1 Corinthian's 11:3

Are You A Controlling Wife
28

At one time in my life I lead my marriage under my own understanding of what I thought was righteous and good. I was all-powerful. God? Who's that? I was rebellious and stubborn to my husband because I was married to my selfish lifestyle and wayward beliefs that kept me from accepting and recognizing God.

I rejected my husband sexually because I often thought all he wanted was sex. How could anyone love me, after all I didn't like the person who I had become? I rejected God for my life too, and that was the biggest mistake I had ever made.

I wanted to be in control just like most women want to be in control of their destiny and their life. And women do control well. In many marriages today women control the ship with poisonous demands while their husband's cringe in the galleys like little lost boys who can't find their way home. This is really happening, folks, and most people take it all in with a grain of salt.

Hollywood filmmakers and the Foreign Press promote and support the woman's movement by slowly creating men to be distorted wimpy guys.

The agenda has been going on for sometime now. It is a slow brainwash movement through the use of Hollywood and TV to make people think it is acceptable to be something other than they truly were meant to be. Whether this is done for political reasons or not, it doesn't matter because it is all in direct rebellion to God of Creation. It is a bunch of propaganda to get people to give in and believe in them instead of God.

Ask yourself this. Did God make another man out of the rib of Adam to be his companion? How could two men make babies and multiply the earth? They would both die old men and creation would be over!! Did God give Eve a penis? Why is woman made with such beauty and sexual care if not to give the "real man" great satisfaction in bed?

Do not lie with a man as one lies with a woman; ...
Leviticus 18:22

When depraved films become highly praised for their outright deviance the world is surely living in Sodom. Ah yes, biblical history coming back alive in the world. It happens all the time. I don't take the bible literally but you don't have to!! Look at the whole theme of the bible and it will answer all the questions any of us may have on morality, values and ethics.

Do you not know that the wicked will not inherit the kingdom of God? Do not be deceived; neither the sexually immoral nor idolaters nor adulterers nor male prostitutes nor homosexual offenders or thieves or the greedy nor drunkards nor slanderers nor swindlers will inherit the kingdom of God.
1 Corinthians 6:9

Why do you think there is so much divorce in this country? Some men are rethinking their own sexuality and deciding to go ahead and give women the lead to direct the ship to shore. They are bowing down to the woman's movement because they have no spirituality, belief and religious conviction within them. They're not the captains of their own ships because they themselves have no captain! This is the root of the problem. Where there is no God, there is no righteousness.

142

This is where you come in. Be the woman for your husband so he can get a taste of knowing what it is like to be under the spirituality of Jesus Christ. God is head of Christ and Christ is head of man and man is head of woman. This is the ideal arrangement for marriage.

So you see, it is not just the woman who needs to submit but also the man. If the man will not submit to Christ, then how can he expect his wife to submit to him? Help your man submit to Christ for your marriage today. When a man does not allow God to command his own life he has no direction for his wife and family and cannot lead his home correctly because his heart does not hold the proper guidance of scripture. There is no spiritual conviction to lead the home. The woman will take advantage of her spiritual bankrupt husband and become out of control thinking she is really in control. She will become bossy, stubborn, controlling and rebellious in the marriage because she has been brainwashed into believing she is superior to her male counterpart. I hope this is not happening in your marriage.

You see the woman's movement consuming Hollywood films all the time. You see it on TV every single night in those ridiculous comedy shows. Women being belligerent in the home, ignoring her children, committing adultery because she wants to have her own career and live the way SHE WANTS. It doesn't matter what God wants for her. She is a desperate housewife/woman? She makes herself desperate! This degrades women, don't you think?

The home only needs proper spiritual guidance to lead it according to its true purpose. To love, honor, respect, and above all *commit* your self to one another. You can get the ball rolling for your marriage by doing those things that you can to help your husband see that your marriage would be better if he applied the rock solid truths of God into it. There is no reason for divorce when we have God.

Understand, I'm not against women, I'm for women, I love them, and I am a woman! But unfortunately it is an unethical philosophy taking over the mind of women today.

It is destroying families. It is appalling how this accepted wisdom from the world is overtaking the minds of both men and women. I believe that if a woman of the home can see clear enough to take her role as wife and mother seriously by acknowledging the spiritual Christ within her soul, she will see the truth for what it is. She doesn't know that the truth will set her free from her self and that the unethical movement she is believing in is in direct rebellion to God and is untruth - a lie told by Satan to break marriages apart.

God made them male and female and said, "For this reason a man will heave his father and mother and be united to his wife, and the two will become one flesh? So they are no longer two, but one. Therefore what God has joined together, let man not separate. Mathew 19:4

She must FIRST fix herself before she can love the man she married properly. She will discover how unique she is of her husband in a good way, and that she can compliment and help buildup her husband rather than constantly battle with him for her missing self. She should not be hesitant to be the beautiful creature God made her to be.

Then they can train the younger women to love their husbands and children, to be self-controlled and pure, to be busy at home, to be kind, and to be subject to their husbands, so that no one will malign the word of God. Titus 2:4-5

Bottom line is marriage is not designed to accommodate two captains. Have you ever seen two captains charting one ship? Have you ever seen two Chief Executive Officers controlling one corporation? Have you ever seen two master chefs in one restaurant? Have you ever seen two dentists in one office? You get my point, right?

If a husband is not the spiritual leader and counsel of the home now, then he desperately needs to become the spiritual leader of the home and take the lead in that arena now! A

Husband ought to accept God for his life, Study the bible diligently, and seek out all that God wants for him and his marriage. A man will never truly be happy until he realizes his purpose and calling in life and then goes after those things with gusto. ♥

Spiritual Cleanse For Your Marriage
29

Often times when we don't feel well, we cleanse the body for physical health to prevent surgery, feel good, look younger, and live longer. What about our spiritual health? Did you know that if we cleanse the mind of unwanted toxins our physical health would also improve? Spiritual cleansing is excellent therapy for negative and destructive emotions, depression, sadness, drug and alcohol addiction, and all other addictions that have to do with the mind and attitude.

Rejuvenate the mind everyday with the positive affirmations of prayer. How can prayer help? The influence of prayer actually gives us the hope, faith, and encouragement that our negative feelings have taken from our heart and mind. I have included this spiritual cleanse in this marriage handbook, because I know that when we have a spiritually clear mind, we are better people. We give more, we love more, and we are more!

Every day we are literally plagued with negative garbage, listening to it, and looking at it, to behaving in destructive ways because of it, and all this upsets the equilibrium of our minds. We become out of whack, out of focus, unable to recognize our marriage in the right light. Have you ever thought that maybe it is all the harmful garbage in the world that brings on depression, addiction, and bad feelings? If we are under control of addiction or depression how can we ever recognize the spiritual aspects of our nature? I know first hand that addiction keeps us far from God. So then how do we not know that all we need is a spiritual cleanse to free us from the grips of what is controlling us?

In other words, is it really a chemical imbalance in the brain, like doctors want us to believe that makes some people depressed or addicted to a substance? And if it is a chemical imbalance, could it have something to do with lifestyle/environment -- whether it's through what a person eats and drinks or other contaminates that are entering their system?

CEO's and business owners use affirmations in their corporations to keep the salesmen positive and optimistic. It is a well-known fact that positive minds sell more products. So then why couldn't a positive mind learn to forgive and love completely too?

Every day prayer not only lets God know that we are genuinely seeking his spiritual counsel but also makes us feel better about who we are, even when we are battling with an addiction or just plain old negative feelings.

That's right, you will not come out of your addiction or negative feelings in a day, or a month, it takes a continual prescribed amount of God in your life everyday to one day realize, "Hey, I don't need to drink to feel good about myself." Or, "I don't need to hide behind my destructive feelings that are ruining my marriage anymore."

Applying prayer into our life is the first step to overcoming the negative aspects of character and supercharging the positive aspects within us. The first thing we need to do is to humble our selves to prayer. We need to remember that we are praying for a reason; a purpose, and not necessarily to get what we want but to get closer to God and become more spiritually aware.

How should we pray? We can pray anytime of the day and anywhere. We do not have to be in Church and we do not have to let others hear our personal prayers to God. We are in control of how, when and what we pray. Prayer begins in the mind and ends in the heart. We can pray silently and God hears us.

Prayer involves humbleness and humility. It entails that we trust that God is listening to us as we pray and that our prayers we'll get answered. But our prayers may not get answered the way we want. Many times prayers are answered in the way that God knows is best for us, not what we think is best for us. Prayer involves talking to God through our prayers, bible study, and recognizing God as our source.

I have put together a one month spiritual cleanse that will help bring you closer to God, your loved ones, and your self using the power of affirmations, and prayer for more positive and spiritual way of thinking for your life.

🕊 🕊 🕊

Week one:
Focus on love. Loving God, being more loving to others, giving of ones self, loving neighbor and self. Be Love!

Prayer:
Love is patient, love is kind. It does not envy, it does not boast, it is not proud. It is not rude, it is not self-seeking, it is not easily angered, it keeps no records of wrongs. Love does not delight in evil but rejoices with truth. It always protects, always trusts, always hopes, always preserves. 1 Corinthians 13:4-7

Affirmation prayer:
God help me to be more loving, humble, forgiving, giving, kind and patient with others and myself. I will strive to Love

God with all of my heart, mind and soul. God is love, and love is God!

Objective:
My objective is to love God first, and then to love myself. To realize that loving God above other things in my life frees me to love others with more of who I am and can become.

Week two:
Focus on wisdom, knowledge, truth and understanding from God. Do NOT seek out wisdom, knowledge, truth, or understanding from culture or society, or from anyone in the world. The bible should be my only source for all understanding and truth.

Prayer:
Who is wise and understanding among you? Let him show it by his good life, by his deeds done in the humility that comes from wisdom. But if you harbor bitter envy and selfish ambition in your hearts, do not boast about it or deny the truth. Such wisdom does not come down from heaven but is earthly, unspiritual, of the devil. For where you have envy and selfish ambition, there you find disorder and every evil practice. But the wisdom that comes from heaven is first of all pure; then peace loving, considerate, submissive, full of mercy, and good fruit… James 3:1317

Affirmation prayer:
God help me to NOT find fault with others, or to be argumentative or judgmental with my spouse, friends, and associates. I will seek your wisdom daily. I will look up the "True" purpose of my situation in the concordance/dictionary of my bible, and allow your wisdom to give me the understanding I need to handle the situation with your divine truth.

Objective:

To gain the understanding that God is my "ONLY" source for everything under the sun for my life and marriage.

Week three:
Focus on my spiritual self by thinking positive and doing constructive things. Take walks outdoors among nature. Try yoga, meditation, or other relaxation techniques to relieve my mind of negative clutter, stress and worry. Take up Pilate's or other non-strenuous exercise to help relieve tension and stress. I know that by doing these things it will reflect back onto my spiritual consciousness. What I allow into my heart and mind reflects back out in my actions.

Prayer:
…To be made NEW in the attitude of your minds, and to put on the New self, created to be like God in true righteousness and holiness. Ephesians 4:23

Affirmation prayer:
God give me the encouragement and strength I need to exist with a renewed attitude of love, giving and forgiving. Help me to put on the new aspects of my personality that I have been hiding within the depths of my soul. Help me to see the good in people even though they are different from me.

Objective:
To recognize the potential within me and to be a new creative, positive person in Jesus Christ, displaying my full potential in everything that I do. To be renewed in mind and spirit. To not focus on my negative feelings of others but to focus more on the positive attributes of my self so I can be more loving and kind to others.

Week four:
Focus on applying God's counsel, love, and wisdom on a daily basis through continual prayer and bible study. Learn to

make God a priority in my life. Make God my habit! Change of heart means change of attitude.

Prayer:
To the man who pleases him, God gives wisdom, knowledge and happiness. Ecclesiastes. 2:26

Affirmation prayer:
God help me to apply your spiritual counsel and wisdom into my daily life to bring me purpose in all that do.

Objective:
To be free from negative and destructive junk, to be the whole and complete spiritual person that I was meant to be and to live life in peace and contentment. Forgive someone today. ♥

Don't Fall Into The Desperate Housewife Trap!
30

What defines a desperate housewife? Would it be a bunch of flighty, sexually desperate married women who hop from bed to bed? Have you noticed how the TV show Desperate Housewives demeans women! Many people might think the show is real cute and funny but what's so funny about a married woman being disloyal to her husband?

A wife of noble character who can find? She is worth far more than rubies. Proverbs 31:10

In the bible day's rubies were more precious than gold, and we all know how precious gold is today. Why do you think it was important to have a noble wife back then? Isn't it important today for a man to be married to a woman of good character? How does it help the man if his wife is a woman of godly character? It builds him up, doesn't it? Husbands aren't so lucky today. It's hard to find a woman who remains pure until marriage.

But this is what happens when women have been conditioned into believing its okay to have a multitude of sexual partners before and even after marriage. They have been told to take

152

their time and experiment, after all there is a lot of fish in the sea, try them all! The conditioning process begins when a girl is barely ten years old. It is part of the culture in America. Most fifteen and sixteen year olds already have had sex. This is what happens when a girl doesn't have a strong spiritual authority (protector) when she is growing up, and this is what happens to a woman who has no spiritual authority (protector) in her life and marriage.

But what about AFTER marriage? What do you think? Is this show and others like it trying to sway young women into believing that it's ok to betray their husbands? Maybe they want women to do that, you know, commit adultery? Does it give women the validation they need to deceive their husbands and become sexually misplaced?

No doubt about it, the characters on the show are desperate for love. But it's not funny, it's not cute, it's not appropriate, and it's not acceptable in the eyes of God. It is absolutely shameful to womankind! A married woman shouldn't want to watch another married woman sleeping around. What gives? Does she not have respect for the man she married? What about herself? Does she not respect herself?

In all truthfulness this show is saying that if a woman is not fulfilled and satisfied being a house wife, maybe she ought to go out and flit about a bit, uh? What do you think? Are you a desperate housewife who needs to go flit about like a lightning bug? There are many ways a woman can become fulfilled and satisfied without committing adultery, believe me. It seems all she really needs is a little bit of love and a whole lot of Jesus.

Your word is a lamp to my feet and a light for my path. Psalm 119:105

Unfortunately, when a woman looks for love out in the world this is what she gets back. So you see the world can't love you, it doesn't know what love is, and it actually wants to gobble you up with it. Don't fall into the desperate housewife trap. It might seem glamorous and sexy because the characters are beautiful, but its complete brainwash, that's all it is and there isn't a bit of good come out of it.

Here is one example of a desperate housewife. In desperation an anxious, unfulfilled, and angry housewife seeks answers for her marriage problems by looking out into the world for her answers. She flips on the TV and there's a show on depicting beautiful, sexy women that are making men out to be little boys who need help going to the bathroom. The resent-filled, desperate housewife is hooked, and finally decides to cheat on her husband.

These women are made out to be impious, calculating, and bossy sexpots who come out seemingly looking superior over men. All of this entices women in today's society because they want to be just like those women, instead of the women they really are. Instead of the women God intended for them to be. You are a beautiful person; don't waste it on over-doing the woman you are, but become who it is that you really, truly are. You will respect and love yourself more in the long run. It is the final freedom from self. No more beating your self up when you are happy to be you.

Here is what I got out of watching only fifteen minutes of that show. That episode I happened to be watching had a lot of rebellion, a lot of resentment, and a whole lot of sexual sin. Add them all together and you got desperate!

Meanwhile the angry and desperate housewife with marriage problems is irritated with her lazy, fat husband. She just wants to be happy and satisfied like the beautiful women she sees on television. She becomes infatuated with all the glamour and beauty.

She truly feels these women are in control of their lives even though they continually deceive their husbands. Eventually the anxious housewife cheats on her husband because she feels it is the only way she will be happy and content. This is how she gets the love she needs, the validation she craves, and the satisfaction she wants.

154

The body was not meant for sexual immorality, but for the Lord, and the Lord for the body. 1 Corinthians 6:13

What this woman should have done, instead of being desperate and confused is look within herself for the answers so she could figure out what might be making her feel desperate? Why does she feel out of control? In essence, until she comes to terms with what is really making her feel unfulfilled, she will continue to look out into the world for validation of self.

Cast all your anxiety on him because he cares for you. 1Peter 5:7

The problem is women aren't defining who they are by placing any importance on their God-given positions and working towards that purpose for their life, but rather looking out into the world where women have no idea what God can do for them and their marriage. Without God there is no spiritual purpose for a woman to work towards in her marriage, and she will become bored and desperate just being a housewife. It's as simple as that.

Ladies, don't fall into the desperate housewife trap. A woman does not need to degrade her self by behaving in desperate ways. She only needs to figure out why she would want to become desperate in the first place. Desperation will lead you nowhere, it will take your soul, and you'll never get it back. You already have all the spiritual tools within your self to become a totally satisfied woman without becoming desperate!

Love the man you married! ♥

How A Husband Should Love His Wife
31

Of course I'm going to write another book called *Love The Woman You Married*. Marriage is a two way street. We cannot kiss our self, we tango together, and that means we have to work on the marriage together. After writing so much about how a woman can love her man, it started to feel a bit unbalanced, and so to end this book, I thought I would add a few words for you men out there who might be reading this book.

So until my next book is finished, I just wanted to share an article I wrote just last week on how a husband should love his wife. Ladies, email me and add anything that you feel I may have missed and I'll add it to the book.

❤ ❤ ❤

Men, what have you done lately to show the woman you married that you love her? Do you take her out to dinner? Maybe you buy her flowers or chocolates? A man likes to do these things for a woman because it's easy and fast. But is your wife really appreciating the flowers and chocolates? In this article I have mentioned a few other useful tricks you can do to show your wife that you love her.

1. Validate the woman you married

A woman needs her man to validate her feelings. I know sometimes this is challenging for you to do, especially if you disagree with something she needs your support on. There is a correct way to do this without being offensive and hurting her feelings.

First of all be understanding of your wife's feelings and then collaborate her on her thoughts and ideas even if they differ from yours. In essence, when you listen to your wife's feelings, without criticizing her, you have essentially given her the validation she needs. Everyone needs validation from time to time; it makes them feel useful and productive individuals. Your wife wants to be useful to you more than anyone else, but if you reject her for any reason, maybe she'll feel that you don't need her.

Try to be more understanding of your wife's feelings. By doing this, essentially you will be respecting the woman you married. Tell her how much you like her decorating style, or how she manages the home, or the way she dresses, or whatever it is that you really find appealing about her and tell her so. Find the things about your wife you really like, be honest and tell her the great things you love about her instead of keeping those feelings inside.

Validation is just another form of how a husband can accept the woman he married. By accepting her for the woman she is it will make her feel safe and secure being your wife. A woman who feels safe and loved will ultimately give more of her self to her man. She will want to be protected if you make her feel confident in your loving embrace.

Ironically, a husband can validate his wife's feelings better when he takes the role of spiritual leader in the home. A man who feels secure in his position is more likely to make his wife feel good about who she is in the marriage. They work better together as a team, accomplishing more for them selves and the marriage.

2. Be more Affectionate with your wife

Hold your wife's hand while watching TV, taking a walk, or driving in the car. Massage her back or feet without asking for anything in return. Your wife likes to be touched and fussed over occasionally, know when that time is by being attune to your wife's feelings, and paying special attention to your wife on those days.

3. Surprise your wife with something totally unexpected

Instead of golfing with your buddies on Saturday, take your wife to a romantic outside lunch if it is summer or fireplace lunch in the winter. Then take her to a romantic comedy matinee movie. Or if you have the money to spend, book a hotel room for the night with a Jacuzzi and enjoy the night together! Your wife will love all this.

Make her a homemade all-occasion card on the computer telling her how important she is to you in your life. Make her feel special. Get creative, draw her a picture, and spend time on creating this card, she will love it that you took the time to make her a card rather than simply buying one from the store. It is the simple things in life that mean the most.

4. Give your wife the whole day off from cooking, children, and house cleaning.

This isn't too hard. On your day off do everything for her. Do all the things she does for you. If you don't know how to cook, order pizza or Chinese food. Let your wife spend the day with her friends shopping or going to lunch, etc. When she comes home give her a back rub, take her shoes off, draw her a hot bubble bath and let her take a long bath. When she comes out from her bath, light the candles, caress her some more and just be there for her all the rest of the evening. Be her loving, romantic and protecting man so she can be the woman God made her to be for you.

5. Appreciate all that your wife does

All of the above will show your wife that you love her and appreciate her for everything that she does. Being understanding of your wife's feelings and needs on a consistent basis will improve the quality of your marriage a great deal. By taking the respective roles that God has designed for each gender will greatly enhance the happiness of your marriage. Be the man of the house so she can be the lady of the house.

Don't ever forget as long as you shall live that you wife likes to be touched and hugged without the pressure of sex looming in the near future. Sometimes the hugging and coddling is more important to her than the actual sex act. Not that she doesn't like to orgasm because she loves to orgasm, but that she wants to know that you love her more than the sex act itself. Hug her and cuddle her and you'll most likely get what you want later.

The most important way to show your love is through your acceptance and validation. Are you the kind of guy that discounts his wife's choices, desires, and needs through invalidation? This kind of behavior will cause all kinds of trouble in the marriage. Let me tell you why.

By invalidating your wife in whatever manner, you have essentially rejected her. She will feel as if her opinions, decisions, and beliefs don't count and shouldn't be regarded with importance. She will hold this within her consciousness and it will come back to haunt you later on in the marriage. This won't be on purpose but mostly because you have hurt her. She loves you and when you invalidate her feelings, thoughts, actions, beliefs, views, and opinions, she gets hurt!

Be good to your woman and she will most likely give you what you want to. It's a two-way street sort of deal, marriage. If you don't dance, she won't either. Make her want to dance with you.

Let me tell you a big secret about woman, which also includes your wife. Your wife may ask you for your opinion on something because it is in her nature to get a second opinion, other than her own, but that does not necessarily mean that she will go with your opinion or your opposing viewpoint.

I'm not talking about the submission thing here either. What I'm talking about is just everyday thoughts and actions of your wife. If for some reason you really feel that it is best that you disagree with her thoughts and feelings, do so AFTER you have said something positive about the way she thinks and feels. Be understanding! If you actually validate her she will see it your way on her own, even if she won't admit it.

Your wife may also like to vent her feelings more then you, not because she needs for you to find a solution so much as just being a sounding board. Please be her sounding board. Let her talk it off her chest. That is how women release some of their energy by talking. You already knew that, right?

Don't forget, give her validation in what she has to say, and then ask her if she is looking for an opinion and or solution first before giving her one. This doesn't make much sense to you, but to us women it makes a lot of sense.

After you have shown your wife how much you love her, then you can buy her the chocolates and flowers. Don't buy her the cheap chocolates either.

Take the time to show how much you love your wife. ♥

Angie Lewis is the author of *Journey on the Roads Less Traveled*, a spiritual memoir about love, life, marriage, addiction, forgiveness and faith. A spiritual journey

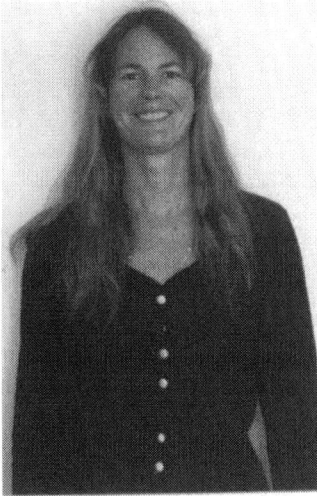

she has revealed to all those who seek out biblical truths for their life.

To learn more about *Journey* or Angie's marriage ministry, Heaven Ministries, visit www.heavenministries.com

Journey on the Roads Less Traveled
http://www.spiritual.journeybooks.4t.com
ISBN 1-4137-8890-4

60529420R00099

Made in the USA
Lexington, KY
09 February 2017